known as factory farms. The lives
are unnatural and unhappy. For ma
breeding and early separation of
partial or total immobilization, lack of fresh air and natural food, and
lack of social interaction with other animals of the same species. The
chapter on the treatment of animals in factory farms makes
uncomfortable reading. As responsible consumers, however, we must
not shut our eyes to the processes by which meat and dairy products
are produced.

A vegetarian diet causes a minuscule amount of environmental
destruction and pollution compared to the amount caused by a diet
that includes animal products. The production of animal products is
a major cause of world environmental pollution and of the destruction
of the world's forests and grasslands.

If you wish to improve your health, if you believe that all creatures
have a right to life without abuse, or if you wish to stop the
environmental destruction caused by producing animal products, it
may be time to change your eating habits.

A note on organically grown food: Food grown organically is better
for human health and causes far less pollution than food grown by
chemical methods.

This book is dedicated with total devotion
to my one and only Angel on earth.
Thank you for your trust, help, support,
love, and affection.

Why Vegetarian?

A Healthy, Humane, and Environmentally Friendly Approach to Food

LYNDA DICKINSON

Gordon Soules Book Publishers Ltd.
West Vancouver, Canada
Seattle, U.S.

Canadian Cataloguing in Publication Data
Dickinson, Lynda, 1955-
  Why vegetarian?

  Includes bibliographical references.
  ISBN 0-919574-89-0

  1. Vegetarianism.   2. Vegetarian cookery.   3. Vegetarianism—
Societies, etc.—Directories.   4. Animal welfare—Societies, etc.—
Directories.   I. Title.
TX392.D52 1994   613.2'62   C94-910722-0

Published in Canada by
Gordon Soules Book Publishers Ltd.
1352-B Marine Drive
West Vancouver, BC V7T 1B5

Published in the United States by
Gordon Soules Book Publishers Ltd.
620-1916 Pike Place
Seattle, WA 98101

Typeset by A.R. CompuType Graphics, Vancouver, BC, Canada
Printed and bound in Canada by Best Book Manufacturers Inc.

Contents

Acknowledgments

Very special thanks to

Gordon Soules, publisher and true gentleman, for having trust in my work and belief in the issue;

Lois Richardson, Gudrun Will, and Sheila Jacobs for many long hours of much-needed work on my manuscript;

Antoinette, my sister, and Massimo, my brother-in-law, for never being too far away to provide love, humor, prayers, and support; and

all the wonderful people I spoke with and wrote to for information for *Why Vegetarian?*

CHAPTER 1

Vegetarian Recipes

Here are some recipes to introduce you to preparing vegetarian food.

Snacks and Appetizers

Italian Bagel Bruschetta *(Lynda Dickinson)*
10 to 16 bagel halves, plain or garlic
¼ cup (60 mL) olive oil
4 ripe medium tomatoes
1 tbsp (15 mL) dried oregano flakes

Place bagel halves on large platter. Using a spoon, drip small amount of olive oil over them.

Slice and dice tomatoes and place in a bowl. Pour remaining oil over tomatoes and let soak for 1 to 2 minutes. Add oregano. Mix well.

Carefully spoon mixture over bagel halves. Sprinkle with dash of oregano flakes and serve. Great as appetizer or snack. Mixture can also be poured over bread or baked potato.

Serves 2 to 4.

Sesame Green Dip *(Ivana Biondich, Redmond, Washington)*

15 oz (425 g) raw sesame butter
juice of 3 whole lemons
1 bunch fresh parsley, stemmed and chopped
2 large cucumbers, chunked
6 celery stalks, chunked
2 large green peppers, chunked
1 tbsp (15 mL) sea salt
5 cloves garlic, crushed
lemon pepper to taste

In food processor or blender, blend sesame butter and lemon juice for 3 minutes. If mixture is too stiff, add up to ¼ cup (60 mL) water.

Gradually add rest of ingredients and blend for 2 to 4 minutes. Chill or freeze. Good veggie dip or topping for baked potatoes.

Soy Pâté *(Ivana Biondich, Redmond, Washington)*

1 cup (250 mL) soy granules (textured soy protein)
1 tbsp (15 mL) sea salt
15 oz (425 g) tomato sauce
½ cup (125 mL) water
1 small bunch parsley, stemmed and chopped
6 small green onions, chopped
5 garlic cloves, minced
2½ cups (625 mL) walnuts, chopped

In medium bowl, mix soy granules, sea salt, and tomato sauce. Add water and mix well. Let soak for 10 minutes.

Add parsley, onions, garlic, and walnuts. Pour mixture into blender or food processor and blend for 2 to 3 minutes. Chill. Serve on bread or crackers. Great as a sandwich spread. Makes six cups.

Eva's Incredibly Edible Pâté *(Eva von Haugwitz, Durham, North Carolina)*

½ cup (125 mL) concentrated vegetable broth
6 oz (180 g) firm tofu
2 carrots, diced
½ onion, diced
4 radishes, diced
1 green pepper, diced
2 green onions, diced
1 Tbsp (15 mL) dill, fresh
2 Tbsp (30 mL) tahini (sesame butter)
paprika to taste
pepper and sea salt to taste
½ cup (125 mL) sunflower seeds
½ cup (125 mL) nuts, ground
½ cup (125 mL) oat bran

In a blender, blend broth, tofu, carrots, onion, radishes, green pepper, green onions, dill, and tahini for 3 minutes or until smooth and semiliquid.

Pour mixture into mixing bowl and add paprika, pepper, salt, sunflower seeds, nuts, and oat bran. Mix by hand for 3 minutes or until smooth and creamy. Serve as a dip with raw vegetables or as a sandwich spread.

Stuffed Grape Leaves *(Ivana Biondich, Redmond, Washington)*

2 cups (500 mL) cooked brown rice
¼ cup (60 mL) olive oil
1 tbsp (15 mL) fresh dill
salt to taste
6 small green onions, finely chopped
1 bunch fresh parsley, stemmed, finely chopped
3 tbsp (45 mL) dried mint leaves, finely crushed
juice of 2 whole lemons
2 cups (500 mL) alfalfa sprouts
¾ cup (80 mL) sunflower seeds

10 pickled grape leaves

Let cooked rice cool for 5 minutes. Combine oil, dill, salt, onions, parsley, mint, lemon juice, alfalfa sprouts, and sunflower seeds. Mix well. Pour onto rice and mix thoroughly.

Using a tablespoon, fill each grape leaf with rice mixture and roll up. Place on platter with seam side down. Chill for 5 to 10 minutes. Great as a side dish or as finger food for parties.

Serves 4 to 6.

Avocado Sandwich *(Ivana Biondich, Redmond, Washington)*
8 slices whole wheat bread, toasted
mustard to taste
8 lettuce leaves
1 firm ripe avocado
1 tomato, thinly sliced
1 green pepper, thinly sliced
1 cucumber, thinly sliced
onion, thinly sliced, to taste
dill pickle slices, to taste
vegan mayonnaise

Spread mustard to taste on 4 pieces of bread. Place one lettuce leaf on each. Slice avocado in half, remove pit, slice into strips, and peel. Place strips of avocado on top of lettuce leaves. Layer tomato, green pepper, cucumber, and onion. Top with remaining lettuce leaves.

Spread vegan mayonnaise on remaining 4 pieces of bread and cover sandwiches.

Serves 2 to 4.

Soups, Salads, and Light Dishes

Better than Chicken Soup *(Roberta Kalechofsky, Jews for Animal Rights, Marblehead, Massachusetts)*

1 lb (450 g) yellow split peas
1 cup (250 mL) parsnips, grated
1 cup (250 mL) carrots, grated
2 bay leaves
salt and pepper to taste

In large pan, cook split peas in water. Halfway through cooking time, add other ingredients and cook until done. Remove from heat and cool for 5 to 10 minutes.

Serves 6 to 8.

Lentil Vegetable Soup *(Stirling Johnson, Madison, Wisconsin)*

7 cups (1.75 L) water or vegetable stock
1½ cups (375 mL) lentils, uncooked
2 potatoes, chopped
2 large carrots, chopped
1 green pepper, chopped
1 large onion, chopped
2 tsp (10 mL) celery seed
2 tsp (10 mL) chili powder
garlic and salt to taste

In large pot, bring water or vegetable stock to a vigorous boil. Add lentils, vegetables, and spices. Lower heat to medium-low and cook uncovered for 45 minutes or until lentils are soft. Serve with bread and salad.

Serves 4 to 6.

Très Belle Salade *(Sheila Clark, Toronto Vegetarian Association, Toronto, Ontario)*

2 medium beets, steamed
½ cup (125 mL) green cabbage, finely cut

½ English cucumber, peeled and sliced
2 medium pieces candied ginger
2 cups (500 mL) dandelion greens
½ cup (125 mL) presoaked raw almonds
2 tbsp (30 mL) raisins
2 tbsp (30 mL) presoaked Arame seaweed
2 tbsp (30 mL) fresh lemon thyme
1 large carrot, chopped
2 tbsp (30 mL) soy or safflower mayonnaise

Steam beets for approximately 20 to 25 minutes. Remove from heat and place under cold water to make them easier to peel. Peel and chill.

Place chopped cabbage and cucumber in large salad bowl. Wipe sugar off ginger and add to bowl. Add dandelion greens, almonds, raisins, seaweed, lemon thyme, carrot, and mayonnaise. Remove beets from refrigerator and carefully slice. Add to salad and toss thoroughly. A very colorful, tasty salad.

Serves 2 to 4.

Taco Salad *(Nola Meeds, Seattle, Washington)*
1½ cups (375 mL) cooked lentils, drained and chilled
1 large head lettuce
2 medium tomatoes
1 small onion (or to taste)
1 14-oz (400-mL) can black olives, drained
2 cups (500 mL) soy cheddar, shredded

Dressing:
1 cup (250 mL) sour cream substitute
1 cup (250 mL) salsa or hot sauce

Cut lettuce, tomatoes, and onion to desired sizes and toss with lentils. In separate bowl, mix sour cream substitute and salsa; pour over salad and mix well. Add olives and sprinkle soy cheddar over top. Serve with fresh tortillas or tortilla chips.

Southern Potato Salad *(Sylvia Warren, Holbrook, New York)*

5 large potatoes
3 small onions, finely chopped
2 tbsp (30 mL) relish
2 tbsp (30 mL) mustard
3 tbsp (45 mL) vegan mayonnaise
1 tbsp (15 mL) garlic powder
2 carrots, shredded
3 tbsp (45 mL) fresh or dry dill weed
salt and black or red pepper to taste
1 red pepper, cut in 8 strips
1 tomato, thinly sliced
¼ cup (60 mL) carrots, shredded

Peel potatoes, place in medium pot, and cover with water. Over medium heat, boil for approximately 15 to 20 minutes or until soft. Drain and cool for 5 minutes. Cut into bite-sized pieces and place in large mixing bowl.

Add onions, relish, mustard, vegan mayonnaise, garlic powder, carrots, dill, salt, and pepper. Mix well.

Spoon into 4 salad bowls. Top each with 2 strips red pepper and 2 slices tomato and sprinkle with remaining shredded carrots. May also be garnished with fresh dill.

Serves 4.

Joyous Pizza *(Julie Hattori, Toronto Vegetarian Association, Toronto, Ontario)*

1 cup (250 mL) brown rice
½ cup (125 mL) millet
3½ cups (875 mL) water
2 oz (30 g) dried tomatoes
14 oz (420 g) tomato paste
2 large garlic cloves, minced
1 tsp (5 mL) oregano
1 tsp (5 mL) basil

15 oz (450 g) whole kernel corn
1 zucchini, thinly sliced

In large pan, soak rice and millet in 3½ cups (875 mL) water for 4 to 8 hours. In large mixing bowl, soak dried tomatoes in water to cover for 2 to 4 hours. Drain.

Place pan with rice and millet mixture over medium heat and bring to a boil; simmer until all liquid is absorbed. Set aside to cool.

Preheat oven to 350°F (180°C).

Grease two 9-inch (23-cm) pie plates and line with a thin layer of rice/millet mixture. Bake the crust for 5 minutes. Cool.

In mixing bowl, mix tomato paste with up to ¼ cup (60 mL) water until it has a spreadable consistency. Add garlic, oregano, and basil. Mix well, and spread mixture onto pizza crusts. Sprinkle corn kernels over mixture. Add zucchini slices and tomatoes.

Bake for 30 minutes. Cool and serve.

Serves 4 to 6.

Pulse Savory *(The Movement for Compassionate Living, Surrey, England)*
¼ cup (60 mL) beans of choice
¼ cup (60 mL) tomatoes, diced
pepper and sea salt to taste
1 tsp (5 mL) yeast extract
herbs of choice
4 tbsp (60 mL) water

In medium pot, soak beans in 2 cups (500 mL) water overnight or for 8 hours.

Over medium heat, bring beans to quick boil. Reduce heat and simmer for 40 to 45 minutes or until well cooked. Add water as required. Drain and cool.

Preheat oven to 350°F (180°C).

Using a potato masher, mash beans until texture is smooth. Place in medium bowl. Mix in tomatoes, pepper, sea salt, yeast, and herbs. If mixture is too thick, add up to ¼ cup (60 mL) water.

Lightly grease a large cookie sheet. Shape mixture into patties and bake for 20 minutes. Great side dish with cranberry applesauce or as a hamburger substitute.

Serves 2.

Nut Mince *(The Movement for Compassionate Living, Surrey, England)*

½ cup (60 mL) onions, chopped *or* 1 tomato, thickly sliced
2 tbsp (30 mL) oil
1 tsp (5 mL) yeast extract
½ cup (125 mL) hot water
⅛ cup (30 mL) porridge oats
salt and pepper to taste
¼ cup (60 mL) grated nuts

In large skillet over medium heat, cook onion or tomato in oil 5 to 8 minutes or until soft.

Stir in yeast extract, hot water, porridge oats, salt, and pepper. Cook for 15 to 20 minutes. Stir in nuts and mix well. Serve immediately as a side dish.

Serves 2.

Potato Roast *(Ida Celli, Downsview, Ontario)*

8 large potatoes, quartered
4 carrots, sliced
2 celery stalks, sliced
½ onion, chopped (optional)
1 vegetable cube
1 cup (250 mL) hot water
1 cup (250 mL) white wine
2 tbsp (30 mL) olive oil

Preheat oven to 350°F (180°C).

Lightly grease a large roasting pan. Place potatoes, carrots, celery, and onion in pan and mix. Dissolve vegetable cube in hot water. Pour water and wine over vegetables. Cover and cook for 55 minutes.

Remove cover, spoon olive oil over mixture, and cook uncovered for an additional 45 minutes or until water in bottom of pan has completely dried. Excellent side dish.

Serves 6 to 8.

Main Courses

All-American Shish Kebabs *(People for the Ethical Treatment of Animals, Washington, D.C.)*

1 lb (450 g) cubed tofu, previously frozen and thawed

Marinade:

½ cup (125 mL) water
½ cup (125 mL) soy sauce
1-inch (2.5-cm) piece fresh ginger, minced
2 tbsp (30 mL) oil
2 tbsp (30 mL) lemon juice
2 tbsp (30 mL) peanut butter
¼ tsp (1 mL) cayenne pepper
1 clove garlic, sliced

Vegetables for kebabs:

2 large green peppers, cut in squares
2 large onions, cut in wedges
12 small, whole button mushrooms
12 cherry tomatoes
1 zucchini, cut in wedges

Before making kebabs, freeze and defrost tofu to change its consistency from soft to chewy.

In large square pan, mix marinade ingredients. Gently press excess water out of tofu and cut into 1-inch (2.5-cm) cubes. Place cubes in marinade, cover, and let soak about 20 minutes, stirring occasionally.

Thread marinated cubes of tofu onto skewers, alternating tofu with vegetables. Place skewers in pan and spoon marinade over them.

Cook on outside grill. Baste occasionally with marinade while turning. Cook for 5 minutes or until vegetables are browned on the edges. Chunks of pineapple may be substituted for vegetables. Serves 4.

Sea Cakes *(Molly Thorkildsen and Will Bonsall, Khadighar, Farmington, Maine)*

4 cups (1 L) water
2 cups (500 mL) cracked oats
½ cup (125 mL) crumbled tempeh
½ cup (125 mL) whole wheat flour
2 tbsp (30 mL) soy flour, raw
1 cup (250 mL) onions, diced
½ cup (125 mL) sunflower meal
2 tbsp (30 mL) toasted seaweed
½ tsp (5 mL) lemon thyme
¼ tsp (1 mL) tarragon
1 tsp (5 mL) salt
1 cup (250 mL) cornmeal

Over medium heat, bring water to a boil in large pot. Add all ingredients except cornmeal. Mix well. Cover tightly, reduce heat, and simmer for 45 minutes. Remove from heat and cool for 25 minutes.

Preheat oven to 400°F (200°C).

Pour cornmeal onto a plate. Shape cooked mixture into patties and place in cornmeal. Lightly bread both sides. Place on large, greased cookie sheet. Bake for 20 minutes or until browned. Serve on buns as hamburger substitute or as a side dish.

Serves 4.

Vegan Miso Gravy Casserole *(Nola Meeds, Seattle, Washington)*

8 cups (2 L) water
6 cups (750 g) elbow noodles
3 cups (750 mL) water
2 tbsp (30 mL) miso
1 medium leek, chopped
1½ cups (375 mL) fresh or frozen broccoli, cut up
4 garlic cloves, chopped
8 oz (225 g) firm tofu, cut up
¼ cup (60 mL) margarine
⅓ cup (75 mL) nutritional yeast
⅓ cup (75 mL) flour

In large saucepan, over medium-high heat, bring water to boil.
Add noodles and lower heat. Cook for 20 to 25 minutes, stirring
occasionally. Remove from heat, drain, and place in large bowl.

In separate pan, simmer miso, leek, broccoli, garlic, and tofu in 3
cups (750 mL) water for 5 to 8 minutes.

In large frying pan, melt margarine and whisk in yeast and flour.

Stir miso mixture into margarine mixture and simmer 20 minutes
or until thick. Pour mixture over noodles and stir carefully.

Miso mixture can also be used as gravy over potatoes or stir-fried
vegetables.

Serves 4 to 6.

Curried Vegetable Burritos *(Denise Ford, Animal Emancipa-
tion, Ventura, California)*

melted margarine or olive oil
2 russet potatoes, thinly sliced
½ red onion, thinly sliced
1 tsp (5 mL) coriander
1 tsp (5 mL) cinnamon
1 tbsp (15 mL) vegetable seasoning powder
1 tbsp (15 mL) minced garlic
1 tbsp (15 mL) curry powder

¼ cup (60 mL) corn, canned
¼ cup (60 mL) peas, canned
1 banana, diced
4 chapatis or whole wheat tortillas (at room temperature)

Sauce:
3 tbsp (45 mL) whole wheat flour
1 tsp (5 mL) sugar
1 tbsp (15 mL) curry powder
4 tbsp (60 mL) water, boiling

Heat enough melted margarine or oil to fry potatoes and onions until soft (about 5 minutes). Add seasonings and stir. Add corn, peas, and banana. Stir gently but consistently until hot. Remove mixture from pan with slotted spoon (to retain seasoned oil). Place equal portions on each of the four chapatis. Roll into burritos, with seam side down. Set aside, and make sauce.

Mix sauce ingredients and dissolve in boiling water. Slowly and carefully stir into seasoned oil left in pan. Cook slowly until thickened. Remove from heat and let stand for 2 to 3 minutes. Pour over stuffed chapatis, and garnish with slices of tomatoes, cucumber, mango, or papaya.

Serves 2 to 4.

Sunflower Seed Veggie Roast *(Leslie Davies, The Happy Nut House, Natural Foods and Vitamins, Surrey, British Columbia)*

1 cup (250 mL) carrots, grated
1 medium onion, finely chopped
1 cup (250 mL) broccoli, finely chopped
1 cup (250 mL) sunflower seeds, raw
1½ cups (375 mL) oatmeal
4 tbsp (60 mL) tomato paste
1¼ tsp (5 mL) seasoning herbs
1 tsp (5 mL) garlic powder
1 tsp (5 mL) curry powder

Preheat oven to 375°F (190°C).

Grease 5-by-8-inch (13-by-20-cm) loaf pan. Combine all ingredients and mix well. Press mixture into loaf pan and bake for 45 minutes to 1 hour. Cool slightly, slice, and serve.

The mixture can also be formed into patties and fried in oil to make vegetarian burgers.

Serves 6 to 8.

Chili con Corn *(Ivana Biondich, Redmond, Washington)*

6 cups (1.5 L) water

1½ cups (375 mL) corn noodles or macaroni

6 to 8 small green onions, diced

1 15-oz (450-mL) can pre-cooked red beans

½ cup (125 mL) soy granules (dehydrated textured soy protein) soaked in ½ cup (125 mL) water for 10 minutes

1 tbsp (15 mL) cumin powder

1 tbsp (15 mL) paprika powder

1 tbsp (15 mL) chili powder

1 tbsp (15 mL) garlic powder

1 tbsp (15 mL) salt

2 small zucchinis, diced

2 green peppers, diced

3 large tomatoes, diced

1 cup (250 mL) corn kernels, canned

Bring water to boil in a large saucepan. Add noodles or macaroni and cook for approximately 7 minutes. Add rest of ingredients and mix well. Cook over low heat just to warm. Don't overcook—crunchy veggies are great!

Serves 4 to 6.

Tofu Parmigiana *(Jo-Ann Murphy, Simply Delicious Natural Health Foods, Pennsville, New Jersey)*

¼ cup (60 mL) red wine vinegar

¼ cup (60 mL) tamari

¼ cup (60 mL) water

2 garlic cloves, crushed

1 tsp (5 mL) dried basil

1 tsp (5 mL) minced parsley

1 tsp (5 mL) black pepper

1 tsp (5 mL) Arame seaweed, crushed

1 lb (450 g) frozen tofu, thawed and well drained

1 cup (125 mL) cornmeal

½ cup (125 mL) sesame oil

2 cups (500 mL) spaghetti sauce

½ lb (225 g) soy mozzarella, thinly sliced

rice or Japanese soba noodles

Preheat oven to 350°F (180°C).

In a large bowl, make a marinade of the vinegar, tamari, water, garlic, basil, parsley, pepper, and seaweed. Mix well and set aside.

Cut tofu into slices ¼ inch to ½ inch (½ cm to 1 cm) thick. Put tofu slices into marinade and let soak for 3 to 4 hours or until marinade is completely absorbed.

Dredge tofu slices in cornmeal until well coated. Heat heavy skillet over medium heat. Add sesame oil and fry tofu slices on both sides until golden brown. Add more sesame oil as needed. Drain tofu on paper towel.

In a shallow baking dish, spoon in enough spaghetti sauce to cover bottom. Arrange tofu slices on top of sauce. Cover with remaining sauce. Place slices of soy mozzarella on top. Bake for 15 minutes or until soy mozzarella is melted. Let sit for 10 minutes. Can be served alone or over boiled rice or cooked Japanese soba noodles.

Serves 4 to 6.

Thanksgiving Bake with Mushroom Gravy *(Ivana Biondich, Redmond, Washington)*

Bread stuffing:

2½ lb (1 kg) potatoes

6 tbsp (90 mL) water or soy milk

pinch salt
1 medium onion, finely chopped
2 cups (500 mL) kale or spinach, chopped
3 carrots, finely diced or grated
3 or 4 celery stalks, finely diced
½ loaf whole wheat bread, cut in bite-sized pieces
1 tsp (5 mL) sage
1 tsp (5 mL) thyme
1 tsp (5 mL) rosemary
1 tsp (5 mL) marjoram
1 tsp (5 mL) paprika
¼ cup (60 mL) sesame seeds
1 cup (250 mL) water

Preheat oven to 375°F (190°C).

Peel potatoes, quarter and boil 20 to 30 minutes. Drain and mash, adding water or soy milk and salt. Set aside.

Combine remaining ingredients and mix well. Put in greased 9-by-10-inch (23-by-25-cm) baking pan. Top with mashed potatoes. Bake for 30 to 40 minutes. Serve with mushroom gravy (see below).

Mushroom gravy:
½ cup (125 mL) oil
½ cup (125 mL) flour
2¼ cups (560 mL) water
6 tbsp (90 mL) soy sauce
⅔ cup (150 mL) nutritional yeast flakes
pinch garlic powder
¼ cup (60 mL) canned mushrooms, sliced

In medium saucepan, combine everything but mushrooms. Cook over medium heat for 5 to 10 minutes until thick, stirring continuously. Stir in mushrooms and heat for 1 minute. Pour over Thanksgiving Bake and serve.

Serves 4 to 6.

Vegetarian Greek Pastitsio *(Kim Bartlett, former editor of The Animals' Agenda, Monroe, Connecticut)*

This is a layered casserole. Use a large baking dish to assemble the two mixtures.

1 30-oz (900-g) box macaroni

Meat-substitute sauce:
2 or 3 onions, chopped
6 tbsp (90 mL) olive oil
1 tbsp (15 mL) oregano, dried
2 tsp (5 mL) basil, dried
1 cup (250 mL) textured vegetable protein
1 14-oz (400-mL) can tomato sauce
¼ cup (60 mL) water
2 tsp (10 mL) cinnamon

Cream sauce:
6 tbsp (90 mL) margarine
pinch salt
pinch pepper
6 tbsp (90 mL) flour
3 cups (750 mL) soy milk
soy parmesan to taste

Cook macaroni according to directions on package. Drain well.

Make meat-substitute sauce:
In medium pan, over medium heat, brown onions in oil. Stir in oregano and basil. Cook for 2 minutes. Add textured vegetable protein and tomato sauce. If mixture is too thick, add water. Cook for 20 to 30 minutes, stirring frequently. Add more water if needed. Stir in cinnamon. Set aside.

Make cream sauce:

In large saucepan, melt margarine. Add salt and pepper. Whisk in flour to make a thick paste. Whisk in soy milk. Stirring constantly, cook mixture 5 to 10 minutes or until thick and creamy. Remove from heat and mix with cooked macaroni; stir in soy parmesan.

Preheat oven to 350°F (180°).

Pour half of the meat-substitute sauce into a large (12-by-15-inch/30-by-37-cm) casserole dish. Pour in half of the macaroni mixture. Repeat layers. Sprinkle soy parmesan to taste over the top and bake for about 45 minutes or until top is golden brown. Cool slightly. Section into squares to serve.

Serves 6 to 8.

Sprouted Grain and Lentil Casserole *(Brynn and Dov Sugarman, Jerusalem, Israel)*

7 cups (1.75 L) water
2 cups (500 mL) whole wheat berries, sprouted
1 cup (250 mL) lentils, brown or green, sprouted
½ cup (125 mL) red lentils, unsprouted
6 carrots, sliced 3 zucchini, diced
½ cup (125 mL) celery, chopped
2 tbsp (30 mL) curry paste or powder (optional)
2 tbsp (30 mL) tamari or soy sauce
2 tbsp (30 mL) tahini (sesame butter)
garlic to taste

Preheat oven to 325°F (165°C).

Put water in large pot. Add berries and lentils (sprouted and unsprouted). Bring to a quick boil. Turn down heat and simmer for approximately 15 minutes or until cooked.

Heat oil in large skillet over medium heat. Add carrots, zucchini, celery, and curry. Mix well. Sauté mixture for 3 to 5 minutes. Remove from heat and add to grain/lentil mixture. Stir in curry, tamari, and tahini. Simmer for 15 minutes more.

Spoon mixture into a lightly greased large
(12-by-15-inch/30-by-37-cm) casserole dish. Bake uncovered for 45
minutes or until top is light brown and casserole is firm in
texture.

Serves 6 to 8.

Cabbage and Potato Simmer *(Sandra Stanton, Farmington, Maine)*

8 to 10 medium potatoes
1 large cabbage
8 tbsp (120 mL) canola oil
2 onions, sliced
3 garlic cloves, diced
½ tsp (2 mL) cumin
½ tsp (2 mL) coriander, fresh
½ tsp (2 mL) dill, fresh
¼ tsp (1 mL) rosemary
salt and pepper, to taste

Over medium-high heat, parboil potatoes about 10 minutes, or
until tender. Drain and cut each potato into 8 even pieces.

Over medium heat, parboil cabbage about 8 minutes, or until
tender. Dice.

Heat canola oil in large pan over medium heat. Stir in onions,
garlic, cumin, coriander, dill, rosemary, salt and pepper. Sauté for
3 to 5 minutes. Add cabbage to sautéed mixture, reduce heat, and
simmer for 10 minutes. Mix well, add potatoes, and heat mixture.

Serves 6 to 8.

Baked Stuffed Zucchini *(Sandra Stanton, Farmington, Maine)*

4 fresh zucchini
4 tbsp (60 mL) canola oil
2 onions, chopped
3 garlic cloves, diced

1 tbsp (15 mL) parsley
½ cup (125 mL) celery, diced
½ loaf whole wheat bread, cut in bite-sized pieces
½ cup (125 mL) raisins
1 cup (250 mL) apple cider
2 tbsp (30 mL) vinegar

Preheat oven to 350°F (180°C)

Cut the 4 zucchini lengthwise. Scoop out centers so that each shell remains about ½ inch (1 cm) thick. Set shells and centers aside and make stuffing.

Sauté onions and garlic in oil in medium skillet over medium heat until golden brown. Add parsley, celery, and zucchini centers. Stir. Add bread and raisins; mix well. Remove from heat. Carefully spoon mixture into zucchini halves and lay in greased baking pan.

In small bowl, mix apple cider and vinegar; slowly pour over zucchini. Bake for 30 minutes or until tops are golden brown and zucchini is tender. Parboiled potatoes may be placed alongside zucchini, sprinkled with salt and pepper, and baked until brown.

Serves 4.

Fried Seitan *(Jo-Ann Murphy, Simply Delicious Natural Health Foods, Pennsville, New Jersey)*

Marinade:
2 tbsp (30 mL) red wine vinegar
2 tbsp (30 mL) tamari
2 tbsp (30 mL) water
½ cup (125 mL) Arame seaweed, crumbled
1 garlic clove, crushed
½ tsp (2 mL) pepper
½ tsp (2 mL) minced parsley
16 oz (450 g) seitan (a wheat starch used in place of meat)
½ cup (125 mL) whole wheat pastry flour
dash pepper

¾ cup (180 mL) soy milk
2 tsp (30 mL) lemon juice
1 cup (250 mL) wheat crackers finely crushed
6 tbsp (90 mL) sesame oil
½ cup (125 mL) onions, chopped
½ cup (125 mL) canned mushrooms, sliced
pinch of sea salt
2 cups (500 mL) soy milk
1 tbsp (15 mL) kuzu (Japanese arrowroot)

Make marinade:
In large mixing bowl, combine marinade ingredients. Cut seitan into ¼-inch (.5-cm) slices. Marinate seitan overnight or for 8 hours.

When seitan is fully marinated, combine flour and pepper in shallow dish. In another dish, combine soy milk and lemon juice. Set both aside.

Spread cracker crumbs in medium platter. Remove seitan from marinade one slice at a time, reserving marinade. Dredge seitan slices, one at a time, in flour mixture. Dip into milk/lemon juice mix and then into crushed crackers. Coat thoroughly.

In large skillet, heat sesame seed oil over medium heat. Fry coated seitan slices (covered) for 5 to 8 minutes or until golden brown. Remove and place on paper towels on a platter; keep warm.

Make gravy. Add onions to skillet and sauté for about 5 minutes or until soft. Stir in mushrooms and salt. Cover and cook over low heat, stirring frequently until mushrooms are soft and onions have browned (approximately 20 minutes).

Add soy milk and marinade to onions and mushrooms; stir for 3 minutes. Dissolve kuzu in water and add to skillet. Stir into gravy until thickened. Add more kuzu or water until desired consistency is reached. Serve gravy over fried seitan.

Serves 4.

Vegetable Curry *(People for the Ethical Treatment of Animals, Washington, D.C.)*

5 medium potatoes, chopped
2½ cups (625 mL) water
1 cup (250 mL) water
1 onion, chopped
½ tsp (2 mL) chili powder or paprika
1-inch (2.5-cm) piece of ginger, finely chopped
1 tbsp (15 mL) turmeric powder
1 tbsp (15 mL) cumin
2 tbsp (30 mL) coriander
2 cups (500 mL) peas, fresh
4 tomatoes, chopped
1 tbsp (15 mL) lemon juice
8 cups (2 L) cooked brown rice

Boil potatoes in water for 15 minutes. Drain and set aside. In separate large saucepan, simmer onion and spices in 1 cup water for 10 minutes. Stir in boiled potatoes, peas, and tomatoes. Cook over medium heat for 15 to 20 minutes or until tender. Sprinkle with lemon juice and serve over brown rice.

Serves 6 to 8.

Shanghai Delight *(Kevin D. Taneda, Mississauga, Ontario)*

8 cups (2 L) water
13 oz (400 g) Shanghai noodles
4 tbsp (60 mL) vegetable oil
2 garlic cloves, minced
1 tsp (5 mL) ginger root, grated
½ cup (125 mL) Shitake (Japanese) mushrooms
1 cup (250 mL) bok choy, chopped
1 cup (250 mL) bean sprouts
½ medium onion, sliced
1 medium tomato, sliced
1 tsp (5 mL) soy sauce

½ tsp (2 mL) lemon juice
4 tsp (20 mL) brown sugar .
¼ cup (60 mL) tomato paste
½ cup (250 mL) tofu, cubed, drained

Boil Shanghai noodles in water for 3 minutes. Remove from heat, cover, and let stand 10 minutes. Drain and rinse in cold water. Set aside.

In large skillet or wok, heat oil over medium-high heat. Brown garlic and ginger together, then add all other ingredients except tofu and noodles. Mix well and cook for 2 to 3 minutes.

Mix in cooked noodles and tofu and cook for another 2 to 3 minutes on medium heat. If mixture sticks to skillet, add up to ¼ cup (60 mL) water.

Serves 4 to 6.

Black Beans with Rice *(People for the Ethical Treatment of Animals, Wahington, D.C.)*

½ cup (125 mL) water
¼ cup (60 mL) onion, diced
½ cup (125 mL) green or red pepper, diced
½ cup (125 mL) mild chili pepper, canned, diced
1 cup (250 mL) tomatoes, fresh or canned, diced
½ garlic clove, crushed
4 cups (1 L) black beans, canned
4 cups (1 L) cooked brown rice

Simmer onion, pepper, chili pepper, tomatoes, and garlic in water for 10 minutes. Add cooked beans and simmer for 15 minutes. If mixture is too thick, add water to keep beans from sticking.

Serve over cooked brown rice. Top with mild Mexican salsa, and garnish with parsley or chopped tomatoes.

Serves 6.

Broccoli/Spinach Bake *(Andrea Pett, Tarzana, California)*

1 10-oz (300-g) package frozen broccoli spears
1 10-oz (300-g) package frozen spinach
6 oz (180 g) onion dip mix
1 cup (250 mL) sour cream substitute or yogurt substitute
2 cups (500 mL) soy mozzarella, shredded

Preheat oven to 400°F (200°C).

Cook broccoli and spinach according to directions on package. Drain and set aside.

In a medium bowl, combine onion dip mix and sour cream substitute or yogurt substitute. Mix well. Add broccoli and spinach and mix thoroughly.

Spread one-third of vegetable mixture in a 9-by-10-inch (23-by-25-cm) greased glass baking dish. Sprinkle with one-third shredded mozzarella. Repeat layers twice more. Bake uncovered for 30 to 40 minutes.

Serves 2 to 4.

Shepherd's Pie Deluxe *(JoAnne Schwab, Canadian Vegans for Animal Rights, Toronto, Ontario)*

1¼ lb (575 g) eggless lasagna noodles
2 tbsp (30 mL) oil
2 onions, chopped
1 broccoli spear, cooked, chopped
1½ cups (375 mL) mushrooms, canned, sliced
1¾ cups (450 mL) peas, canned
1¾ cups (450 mL) corn, canned
1¾ cups (450 mL) beets, canned, with juice
6 large potatoes, cooked
¼ cup (60 mL) soy milk
¼ cup (60 mL) oil
¼ tsp (1 mL) sea salt
½ cup (125 mL) tomato sauce
paprika

Preheat oven to 350°F (180°C).

Cook lasagna noodles. Drain and set aside.

Sauté onions in oil. Add broccoli; after a few minutes, add mushrooms. Stir and cook for 2 minutes until semisoft. Put sautéed vegetables in large bowl. Mix in peas, corn, and beets. Set aside.

Mash potatoes, adding soy milk, oil, and sea salt. Set aside.

Using six lightly greased individual-sized (approximately 4-by-6-inch/10-by-15-cm) casserole dishes, place one or two cooked lasagna noodles on the bottom of each dish to fully cover bottom. Add half the vegetable mixture. Cover vegetable layer with more noodles. Add one more layer of vegetable mixture and cover with noodles. Spread thin layer of tomato sauce on noodles, and top with a layer of mashed potatoes.

Cook uncovered for one hour or until potato layer is golden brown. Cool for 5 to 10 minutes. Sprinkle with paprika and serve in same casserole dishes.

Serves 6.

Desserts

Bara Brith (Traditional Welsh Fruitcake) *(Jo-Ann Murphy, Simply Delicious Natural Health Foods, Pennsville, New Jersey)*

1 lb (450 g) mixed, dried fruits, unsulphured, chopped
1¼ cup (300 mL) fresh brewed Kukicha tea
1 cup (250 mL) Sucanat (sugar-cane sugar), firmly packed
2 oz (60 g) tofu
½ cup (125 mL) soy milk
⅓ cup (75 mL) sweet rice syrup
3 tbsp (45 mL) orange marmalade
2 tsp (10 mL) cinnamon
2¾ cups (700 mL) whole wheat pastry flour
1 tbsp (15 mL) baking powder

Place fruit in a large bowl and pour in tea. Add Sucanat and mix well. Cover and let stand at room temperature overnight or for 8 hours.

Preheat oven to 325°F (170°C). In small pot, bring tofu to a quick boil in 2 cups (500 mL) water. Remove from heat and drain well.

Process tofu in food processor until smooth. Slowly add soy milk and continue processing until texture is creamy smooth. Add tofu mixture to soaked fruit. Stir in rice syrup, marmalade, and cinnamon. Add flour and baking powder and stir until well combined.

Grease, flour, and line with wax paper a 9-by-5-by-3-inch (23-by-13-by-8-cm) loaf pan. Pour dough into loaf pan. Bake for approximately 2 hours, until cake is brown and crusty and toothpick inserted in center comes out clean. Cool approximately 15 minutes before removing from pan.

Serves 6 to 8.

Yam Pie *(Ivana Biondich, Redmond, Washington)*

1⅔ cups (400 mL) Grapenuts cereal
½ cup (125 mL) water or soy milk
4 lbs (2 kg) yams, steamed till soft, peeled, and cut in 1-inch (3-cm) rounds
½ cup (125 mL) fruit concentrate OR ¼ cup (60 mL) honey
1 tsp (5 mL) pumpkin spice mix

For crust, combine cereal and water or soy milk and mix well. (Add more liquid for a softer crust.) Press into lightly greased pie pan, covering sides and bottom evenly. Place under broiler for 1 minute to set.

In food processor, blend yams, fruit concentrate, and pumpkin spice mix for 1 minute or until smooth. Pour into pie shell. Chill for 20 to 30 minutes. Serve with vanilla non-dairy ice cream.

Serves 4 to 6.

Eggless Chocolate Cake *(Nazen Merjian, Manitoba Animal Alliance, Winnipeg, Manitoba)*

2 cups (500 mL) whole wheat flour
1 cup (250 mL) sugar
½ cup (125 mL) cocoa or carob powder
2 tsp (10 mL) baking soda
¼ tsp (2 mL) salt
2 tsp (10 mL) vanilla
1 cup (250 mL) water
1 cup (250 mL) eggless mayonnaise (not tofu mayonnaise)

Preheat oven to 350°F (180°C).

In large mixing bowl, sift and combine flour, sugar, cocoa or carob, baking soda, and salt. Set aside.

In small bowl, combine vanilla, water, and mayonnaise. Mix well and pour into dry ingredients. Mix until thick and creamy.

Lightly grease a 9-inch (23-cm) spring-form pan. Pour in mix and bake for 35 to 45 minutes.

Golden Dreams French Toast *(Ann Myette-Spence, Golden Dreams Bed and Breakfast, Whistler, British Columbia)*

2 cups (500 mL) liquid egg substitute
½ tsp (2 mL) rum flavoring
1½ cups (375 mL) soy milk
cinnamon
8 slices wholewheat raisin bread (thickly sliced)
raisins
walnuts

Combine egg substitute, flavoring, soy milk, and a few shakes of cinnamon. Beat until smooth.

Dip bread slices in mixture and fry in non-stick pan, turning over once, until golden brown. Remove from pan, sprinkle with raisins or walnuts, and serve immediately. Delicious for breakfast or late-night dessert.

Serves 4.

Raw Cranberry Applesauce *(Ivana Biondich, Redmond, Washington)*

2 cups (400 mL) unprocessed frozen cranberries
2 sweet red apples, cored and quartered
½ cup (120 mL) fruit concentrate *or* ¼ cup (60 mL) honey
¼ tsp (1 mL) pumpkin spice mix

Purée ingredients in food processor, using blade, for 2 to 4 minutes. Chill. Serve as topping for vegan ice cream. Also good as side dish.

Note: Foods made with honey taste better the next day.

Tropical Island Fruit Smoothie *(Kevin D. Taneda, Mississauga, Ontario)*

2 large bananas
2 cups (500 mL) vanilla soy milk or rice cream
8 ice cubes
1 tsp (5 mL) brown sugar (optional)

Mix all ingredients in blender for approximately 1 minute or until consistency is thick and creamy. For extra thickness, add ½ more banana. Pour into tall glasses.
Serves 2.

The following fruit combinations may be used:
1 banana and ½ cup (125 mL) fresh or frozen strawberries
1 banana and 1 large persimmon, pitted and quartered
1 banana and 2 kiwi fruits, peeled and halved
1 banana and ½ cup (125 mL) fresh or frozen pineapple
1 banana and ½ cup (125 mL) chunked papaya
1 banana and. . .whatever you like

CHAPTER 2

Vegetarianism for Good Health

"[M]ostly plant foods, and a generous variety of plant foods, . . .
is the kind of diet that is most likely to be associated
with reduced risk of the kinds of diseases
that tend to kill us in this country."
- *Dr. T. Colin Campbell, nutritional biochemist,*
Cornell University

Although many people adopt a vegetarian diet out of ethical concern for animals and the planet, they are also doing themselves a favor. People who adopt a well-balanced vegetarian diet gain great health advantages. Each year millions of people in the Western world are affected by heart failure, stroke, cancer, and other diseases associated with the consumption of animal products—meat, fish, seafood, eggs, and dairy products. A vegetarian diet puts one at lower risk of experiencing coronary artery diseases, high blood pressure, some forms of cancer, and obesity.[1] It also eliminates ingestion of the antibiotic residue and pesticides in animal products; animal flesh is estimated to contain about fourteen times as much pesticide residue as plant food.[2]

Heart attacks are the major cause of death in the Western world. People who suffer heart attacks often have high cholesterol levels. Cholesterol accumulates on the inside walls of the coronary arteries and eventually impairs the flow of blood to the heart, thus causing a heart attack. Animal products contain large amounts of cholesterol, saturated fats, and concentrated protein, all potentially harmful to the human system. To prevent or control heart attacks, medical professionals now advise people to drastically reduce or, even better, completely eliminate animal products from their diet. Even lean meat contains dangerously high levels of fat.[3] Foods derived from plant sources contain no cholesterol, and scientific evidence shows that the high fiber content of a vegetarian diet even helps remove excess cholesterol from the body.[4]

Scientific studies show that the average American male has a 50 percent chance of dying of a heart attack, while the average vegetarian American male has only a 4 percent chance of dying of a heart attack.[5] According to Dr. William Castelli, Director of the Framingham Heart Study, vegetarian men outlive other men by about six years, on average. Dr. Neal Barnard of the Physicians' Committee for Responsible Medicine observes that in Asian countries where the traditional diet contains little meat, heart disease and stroke are much less common than in the West. The exception is affluent classes that have adopted Western dietary habits. Dr. Barnard believes that good vegetarian eating practices should be taught to children at an early age, because heart disease begins in the teenage years: if children are fed animal products, they are trained to prefer these foods, and their control over their health is largely taken away.

More and more studies indicate that there is a link between the consumption of animal products and cancer of the colon. Meat passes through the human intestine very slowly. In order to digest the meat, the liver secretes large amounts of bile acids into the intestine. One of these acids, deoxycholic acid, is converted into a cancer-causing agent. Meat eaters invariably have far more deoxycholic acid in their intestine than do vegetarians, which is one reason they have a higher rate of colon cancer.[6]

Dietary fat also contributes to cancer of the breast, Dr. Barnard says. This type of cancer is almost unheard of in countries such as China and Japan, where little meat is eaten. In North America, one woman in ten develops breast cancer. Cancer of the uterus, ovaries, cervix, and prostate are also attributed in part to dietary fat. Dr. Barnard asserts that 90 percent of cancer is preventable by taking two simple steps: avoiding tobacco and eating a low-fat, non-animal-based diet.[7]

A study of the Hunzakut people of West Pakistan found that these people are completely free of cancer. These people's diet consists mainly of whole grains, such as wheat, barley, and buckwheat; leafy green vegetables; potatoes and other root vegetables; peas and beans; and fruits, chiefly apricots and mulberries.[8]

People who avoid meat, fish, seafood, eggs, and dairy products tend to avoid being overweight and thus avoid the health risks of being overweight. A vegetarian diet is naturally low in fat and calories.

Animal products provide a highly concentrated form of protein. Medical experts now believe that too much protein is detrimental to human health. When a high level of protein is consumed, the kidneys have to work harder than usual. The extra strain is usually not a problem in young people, but in older people, overworked kidneys create health problems.[9] The recommended daily allowance of protein, set by the Food and Nutrition Board (U.S.) is 2 ounces (56 g) per day for men and 1 3/4 ounces (50 g) per day for women. Vegetarians can easily meet these recommendations, as almost all vegetables, seeds, grains, nuts, and beans contain protein.

Humans Are Not True Carnivores

The human species did not evolve as carnivores, or meat eaters. Many scientists believe that when the usual human food of fruits, vegetables, and nuts disappeared during the last Ice Age, people began eating the flesh of animals in order to survive. In Arctic cultures, the practice continued as the only means of survival. In other cultures, it continued simply because humans acquired a taste for meat.[10]

Human anatomical structures differ from those of carnivores. As the eighteenth-century botanist Karl von Linné noted, "Man's structure, external and internal, compared with that of other animals, shows that fruit and succulent vegetables constitute his natural food." Carnivores such as wolves, hyenas, lions, and cats, have distinct anatomical characteristics suited to their diet. For example, they have large mouths, dynamic jaws, and long canine teeth to pierce and tear at raw muscular flesh. Carnivores secrete acid-based saliva suitable for breaking down flesh protein. They swallow their food in large, torn pieces, and practically all of it is digested in the stomach. Their digestive systems secrete an abundance of hydrochloric acids in order to digest tough animal tissue, fur, and bones.

On the other hand, the higher primates, including humans, have small mouths and incisor teeth that are appropriate for biting into fruits and vegetables. They have well-developed flat molars designed to grind and chew grains and nuts. Their jaws, which are not hinged and fixed like those of meat-eaters, are able to move sideways and up and down.[11] Humans secrete alkaline-based saliva, which is better for breaking down and pre-digesting starch in the mouth.

Dr. Neal Barnard explains: "We are quite different from carnivorous animals. Natural carnivores have a digestive tract proportionately about one-fourth as long as that of vegetarian animals. The long, intricate, winding human digestive tract is ill-suited to digesting and expelling flesh food (which decomposes quickly). Among other physiological differences, we have no claws for tearing flesh, but rather an opposable thumb and dexterous fingers which evolved for picking fruit, leaves, grasses, berries, etc. . . . Like all other vegetarian animals, our skin has millions of pores, allowing us to perspire freely to regulate our temperature. Carnivores . . . can't perspire and must pant to cool down. Small wonder that a carnivorous diet gives us so many problems."

Health Risks Caused by Factory Farming
In North America and in many European countries, almost all meat and dairy products come from animals that have been raised in factory farms. In addition to the general health risks of eating meat, eating meat produced in factory farms subjects people to various additional health risks, including the risk of eating the flesh of diseased animals.

In chickens, for example, the most common serious disease is cancer, of the heart, lungs, kidneys, or ovaries. In some cases, it kills the bird, but often the disease is not discovered until slaughter time or in the packing plant. In many cases, only the diseased organs are thrown away; the rest of the animal's body is salvaged for pet food or human consumption.[12]

In intensive factory farms, many of the chickens that die go unnoticed by the stock people. The carcasses are pecked at and half eaten by the surrounding aggressive and frustrated birds. The remains are trampled upon and eventually decompose into the manure floor. These carcasses may harbor bacteria such as salmonella and listeria, which can be passed on to the chickens that eat the carcasses. Salmonella caused more than two thousand cases of food poisoning in the United States in 1990.[13] In the United Kingdom, millions of cases of salmonella food poisoning occur every year.[14] The cases of poisoning from salmonella strains linked most closely to eggs and poultry rose by 25 percent between 1989 and 1990.[15] Many salmonella strains develop resistance to the antibiotics fed to animals, thus making it more difficult to treat that illness in humans who consume the meat of those animals. The Centers for Disease Control, Atlanta, Georgia, which reported these findings, said that cooking the meat is not a certain safeguard against resistant varieties of salmonella.[16]

The conditions of the growth buildings provide a breeding ground for Campylobacter, a bacteria that, according to the Veterinary Record, is "the predominant cause of enteritis (a stomach disorder) in the United Kingdom," and "there is increasing evidence of an association between Campylobacter enteritis and the consumption of poultry meat."[17] The same situation can be assumed to exist in North America.

Pharmaceutical Farming: Drugs in Animal Products
Routine administration of antibiotics and drugs is necessary to combat the many illnesses and diseases associated with excessively overcrowded conditions, poor ventilation, and lack of fresh air. Confined calves are given up to five times more medication than calves raised without confinement.[18] The veal industry in Canada tells consumers "drug withdrawal periods are prescribed for all medication prior to slaughter."[19] However, a report published by the Humane Society of the United States says it is not known "what a safe amount of drug withdrawal time" is to ensure that the calf's system is cleared of drugs prior to slaughter.[20] In addition, the drugs approved for use in calves by the Food and Drug Administration (U.S.) have been tested and approved only for calves allowed to eat solid food, not for formula-fed calves.[21]

A 1988 study of drug residue in meat discovered that formula-fed veal had a 3.2 percent violation rate of antibiotic residue, which is almost three times higher than the percentage found in the meat of veal calves not raised on formula. Such residues pose a risk to people who are sensitive to them and contribute to the development of resistant strains of bacteria. Although the veal industry states that veal is tested for drug residue,[22] only a small percentage of the animals' carcasses are actually inspected.

A study conducted in 1979 found that there are at least 143 drugs and pesticides likely to leave residue in meat and poultry.[23] Of these drugs, "40 are known to cause or are suspected to cause cancer, 18 of causing birth defects, and 6 of causing mutations, but only 46 are monitored by the U.S. Department of Agriculture."[24] The study noted that an estimated 1.9 million tons of beef and 1.1 million tons of swine containing illegal chemical residue were sold to the public in 1976. There are no indications that the situation in Canada and the U.S. has changed since then. Sample testing for drug residue is so minimal that the amount of residue in most meat today is unknown. For example, of almost 3 million cattle slaughtered in 1988, only 263 were tested for traces of Zeranol, an anabolic steroid routinely given to beef cattle. Of 419,122,826 poultry birds slaughtered, only 155 were tested for anti-salmonella sulfa residue.[25]

Although the U.S. Department of Agriculture and Agriculture Canada perform tests to detect chemical residue in meat, tests for chemicals in food take so long to perform that by the time violation levels of chemicals have been detected, most contaminated meat has already been taken to market and sold.

Many different drugs are given to animals raised for human food. The selection depends on the species involved and the wishes of the producers. One substance routinely administered to animals is arsenic, which is used as a growth stimulant for poultry. Pesticides are given to food animals to control parasites and insects in manure piles. Hormones such as progesterone and testosterone are used as growth promoters in animals that have difficulty gaining weight because of high levels of stress and anxiety.

Nitrofurans and Synovex-H, used for heifers, though claimed to be safe, are highly suspected of being carcinogens in humans. This may explain why cancer of the bowel is the second most common cancer in North America and in European countries, where meat is the primary source of protein, and occurs very seldom in countries such as India and Pakistan, where people are predominantly vegetarian.[26]

Antibiotics are used to improve feed efficiency, to increase weight gain, and to prevent or treat disease.[27] They are necessary to control the spread of contagious diseases, such as bovine tuberculosis and diphtheria, which occur where large numbers of animals are closely confined. Antibiotic residue in the meat of factory-farm animals is known to affect the human immune system. In addition, antibiotics routinely added to animals' feed to prevent possible bacterial disease or to promote weight gain and to increase feed efficiency may be responsible for "contributing to the growth of resistant strains of bacteria which cause disease in humans as well as animals."[28] If the overuse of antibiotics in general becomes too widespread, "virulent strains of bacteria that don't respond to antibiotics will spread through the population. Salmonella poisoning, for instance, has become difficult to treat in recent years because the bacteria is often resistant to common antibiotics."[29]

Penicillin is used extensively in raising poultry and to a lesser extent in raising swine. Due to the constant, routine use of penicillin in animals, 25 percent of H-Influenza in humans no longer responds to it. Streptomycin is used as an animal growth promoter, even though it is believed that this antibiotic is responsible for causing kidney and neurological problems in humans. Terramycin is also used as a growth promoter, and it is the most commonly used anti-bacterial drug in animal feed for cattle, poultry, and swine. The antibiotic Virginiamycin is used to promote growth and to prevent dysentery in swine.[30] Food animals often receive additional unmonitored amounts of drugs and chemicals when, in order to reduce feed costs, producers recycle the animals' own excrement by mixing it with regular feed.[31]

Producers claim that if an animal has been taken off the drugs a certain period of time before slaughter, there is little or no danger of there being drug residue in its flesh. This means that sufficient time must elapse between the last dose of the drug and the time of slaughter. Health officials, however, have expressed concern that producers may not always adhere to proper withdrawal periods and that the rules may not always be followed.[32] Because we cannot know the amounts of drug residue or the frequency of its occurrence in meat, eating animal products would mean eating unknown quantities of unidentified drugs.

Choosing a Vegetarian Diet

Dr. Michael Klaper, an anesthesiologist who is a vegan, declares that "there is nothing in animal products that we need to survive." Why not give up the high-fat, high-cholesterol, high-protein, low-fiber diet that is associated with many diseases? By choosing a vegetarian diet instead, you will be making a sound commitment to animal welfare, to your health, and to the survival of the planet.

As more people are becoming aware of the link between the consumption of animal products and life-threatening illnesses and the cruelty and environmental destruction caused by the production of animal products, vegetarianism is gaining in popularity. We have the power to persuade and reform simply by exercising our choice of purchase. Eliminating animal products from your diet is the most effective contribution you can make towards reducing animal suffering and helping our ailing planet.

To make the transition safely and successfully, do it in the way that works best for you. To begin with, you can use the recipes in this book. Then you may want to buy a vegetarian cookbook. Many vegetarian cookbooks provide information on alternatives to meat, dairy products, and other animal products. Specialty vegetarian cookbooks for pregnant women and for people on restricted diets are also available. You may wish to borrow some vegetarian cookbooks from the library first, to see which ones appeal to you most.

Nutrition and the New Four Food Groups
Professionals knowledgeable about both nutrition and vegetarianism are now recommending eating food from what they have classified as the New Four Food Groups.[33]

In April 1991, the Physicians' Committee for Responsible Medicine (PCRM) unveiled a proposal to replace the old Basic Four Food Groups, which have been recommended by the U.S. government since 1956. This revolutionary dietary change was introduced by PCRM president Neal Barnard, M.D., after documenting scientific evidence supporting a low-fat, vegetarian diet as being the regimen most effective at reducing the risk of heart disease, cancer, and obesity.[34] Further studies are under way as a preliminary step to government approval. The New Four Food Groups were also introduced by Denis Burkitt, M.D., the physician who discovered the value of fiber in the diet; T. Colin Campbell, Ph.D., of Cornell University and head of China Health Study, on nutritional factors in health; and Oliver Alabaster, M.D., director of the Institute for Disease Prevention of George Washington University.

PCRM nutritionist Virginia Messina, M.A. (Public Health), states: "The meat and dairy groups were the principal sources of cholesterol and saturated fat, which is the biggest culprit in raising blood cholesterol. These foods are simply not necessary in the human diet." The New Four Food Groups plan does not exclude all other foods; it prescribes only the center of the diet. It shifts the emphasis from a diet centered on animal products to one centered on plant foods.

The old four food groups are meat (at the top of the chart), dairy, grains, and fruits and vegetables. The New Four Food Groups are whole grains (at the top of the chart), vegetables, legumes, and fruits. Foods such as nuts, sweets, dairy products, and meat are considered optional, as they are not required for good nutrition.

What's in the New Four Food Groups?

- **Whole Grains**
  Pasta, bread, cereals, corn, millet, barley, bulgar, buckwheat, and tortillas. Grains are rich in fiber, protein, zinc, B vitamins, and complex carbohydrates. It is recommended that each meal be centered around a grain dish. Recommended daily servings: five or more.

- **Vegetables**
  Dark green, leafy vegetables such as broccoli, kale, spinach, bok choy, and chicory are all packed with nutrients. They are rich in vitamin C, beta-carotene, riboflavin, and other essential vitamins. Dark yellow and orange vegetables such as carrots, winter squash, sweet potatoes, and pumpkin provide extra beta-carotene. Recommended daily servings: three or more.

- **Legumes**
  Beans, peas, lentils, chick peas, baked and re-fried beans, soya milk, tofu, tempeh, peanuts, and peanut butter are all good sources of fiber, protein, iron, calcium, zinc, and B vitamins. Recommended daily servings: two or more.

- **Fruits**

   Fruits are rich in vitamin C, beta-carotene, and fiber. Strawberries and citrus fruits such as oranges, tangerines, and grapefruits are especially rich in vitamin C. Recommended daily servings: three or more.

   For complete nutritional information on the New Four Food Groups, contact:

   Physicians' Committee for Responsible Medicine
   P.O. Box 6322
   Washington, D.C. 20015

CHAPTER 3

Vegetarianism for the Benefit of Animals

"Intensive-raised farm animals undoubtedly suffer
severe stress because they're unable to express
their natural behavior."
—*Stephanie Brown, president of the Canadian
Federation of Humane Societies*

"Never before in human history have the animals that
bring meat to the table been subjected to such cruelties
as in present factory procedures."
—*Professor George Wald, Nobel Laureate and professor
of biology, Harvard University*

Hens and Chickens As Sources of Meat and Eggs

Chickens are social animals with a strong sense of territory. Each bird
has a place in the pecking order and is well aware of its position in
relation to the others. A mother hen will furiously protect her young
chicks against predators and shelter the threatened chicks under her
wings.

Chickens raised on factory farms, however, whether in egg-laying
batteries or in chicken-meat growth buildings (broiler sheds), are treated
as objects rather than animals with sensitivities and capabilities. As
the chickens exist only to produce food for human consumption, the
industry cuts corners to produce as much as possible for as little cost
as possible.

Chickens in factory farms become bored and aggressive and tend
to peck and injure each other. During the chickens' first week of life,
their beaks are cut off to reduce the severity of the injuries and the
incidence of cannibalism. In de-beaking, almost half the beak is cut
off with a hot blade under a guillotine-like pressing machine. The
experience is so traumatic that many chicks die immediately from
shock. Farmers often make mistakes during the procedure and cut off

part of the chicks' tongues and burn their faces. Because anesthetics and analgesics would cause added expense, they are not used. Debeaking deprives chickens of the ability to groom themselves and preen, practices essential for controlling parasites, and can cause difficulties with eating and drinking.

Chickens are bred specifically for either eggs or meat. Because male chicks in the egg industry are not required for egg production, they are killed at birth. Immediately after hatching, the male chicks are either gassed, mashed alive in meat grinders and mixed with food for other animals, or dropped into garbage bins, where they suffocate.[1] The Humane Farming Association of San Francisco, California, estimates that 240 million male chicks are killed annually in the United States—about 656,000 a day. No one can know for certain the degree of pain and anguish endured by these sentient creatures.

Chickens As Egg-Laying Machines
There are about 250 million egg-laying chickens in the United States, 23 million in Canada, and 47 million in the United Kingdom. These hens spend most of their lives in crowded wire-bottomed cages where they cannot stretch their wings and are hardly able to move.

The hens, which have been genetically manipulated in order to be more efficient egg layers, are forced to produce eggs not on their own natural timetable but according to the demands of the factory farm. All aspects of their lives, including the amount of light they receive, their food intake, and their molting times, are controlled artificially. A flock of chickens is treated as a unit, not as a group of individual birds with varying cycles and needs.

Battery cages designed for egg-laying hens on factory farms are small and uncomfortable. The average size is about 10 by 20 by 14 inches (25 cm by 50 cm by 35 cm). The hens kept in these cages have a wing span of 30 to 32 inches (77 cm). Even one hen would have only enough room to stretch one wing at a time, which is cruel enough, but up to five birds are kept in a single cage. They can hardly move at all. Because they are so tightly packed together in one cage, often they must climb over one another to reach food and water. The weaker birds are trampled on and may be crushed to death or may lose the will to live and die of starvation. "Hens do not grow accustomed to cramped living quarters. Given a choice in an experiment, hens that have been kept in small cages for three months avoid such cages more strongly than do hens with less experience of confinement . . . there is no acclimatization or adjustment, but rather a gradual build-up of negative effects as the restriction continues.''[2] This was the conclusion reached in a study by Dr. Marion Dawkins, of Somerville College, Oxford, and Dr. Christine Nicol, of the University of Bristol.

Battery cages are made of wire on all sides. The wire damages the hens' bodies, particularly their feet and legs. Many hens suffer painful malformations of the feet and legs from standing on the wire bottoms of the cages. Because it is difficult for the hens to move around, it is not unusual for a hen's long claws to grow completely curled around the cage wire, thus trapping the hen. If unnoticed by the factory-farm workers, the hen will either starve or be trampled to death by other hens.[3] Constant rubbing against the wire sides of the cage results in loss of feathers and severe damage to the hens' wings and tails. Abscesses form, and the raw and pus-filled areas are pecked at by stronger, more aggressive hens.

The cages are absolutely bare, without nest boxes, perches, or anything for the hens to scratch. The hens are unable to perform their instinctual activities. Boredom leads to head flicking, a compulsive, repetitive behaviour not seen in free-range hens. Frustration and crowding cause the hens to pluck out their own feathers and peck aggressively at each other. In many cases, cannibalism occurs.

The arrangement of the cages invites neglect of the birds. Battery cages in factory farms are stacked up to five tiers high, in long rows. Up to 25,000 birds may be housed in a single building, with as few as three attendants responsible for overseeing them.[4] Proper care of the hens is impossible, as the attendants have difficulty even seeing when the hens in the top and bottom tiers are in distress.

Droppings accumulate in collecting trays underneath each row of cages. When the collecting trays are full, they are automatically scraped and the droppings pushed into a holding pit. Once the holding pit is full, a scraper pushes the huge amount of droppings out of the building. In addition to the discomfort caused by the cage itself, hens on the lower tiers are splattered with the excrement of hens on the upper tiers when it splashes through the wire sides.

Laying eggs is, of course, a natural biological function of the hen. However, hens in battery cages are subjected to what Konrad Lorenz describes as "the worst torture" when laying eggs because they are not able "to retire somewhere for the laying act. It is truly heart-rending to watch how a chicken tries again and again to crawl beneath her fellow cage mates, to search there, in vain, for cover. Under these circumstances, hens will undoubtedly hold back their eggs for as long as possible. Their instinctive reluctance to lay eggs amidst the crowd of cage mates is certainly as great as the one of civilized people to defecate in an analogous situation."[5]

When the egg is laid, the hen's "vent" becomes red and moist and attracts the attention of aggressive, frustrated, and bored cage mates who peck at this sensitive spot on weaker birds. This often leads to fights and general pecking at each other's feathers. The pecking causes blisters and infection. Continual pecking results in feather loss. These displays of aggression are often followed by bouts of self-mutilation.

To decrease aggression, producers keep the buildings in partial or total darkness, except at feeding times. The darkness gives the hens a false sense of night and makes them believe it is time to sleep.

Molting, when birds lose their feathers and temporarily cease laying eggs, occurs naturally on average once a year, at different times for different hens. In the factory farm, however, whenever egg production declines, a "force-molt" period is imposed on the entire stock to reduce the loss of income from lowered egg production. Forced molting is brought about by withholding food for about seven days and water for up to four days, thus shocking the hens' systems into an unnatural loss of feathers. Forced molting lasts for approximately six weeks. Up to 25 percent of caged hens do not survive forced molting. As food is reintroduced and slowly increased, the surviving hens begin to grow new feathers. Soon after, the entire stock begins another cycle of continual egg laying.[6] Forced molting has been forbidden in the U.K. since 1987.

The normal life span of chickens under natural conditions is between four and eight years. By the time caged laying hens have produced eggs for eighteen months, their productivity has decreased. Once they are no longer profitable, they are sent to slaughter.

Chickens Raised for Meat

Every year, approximately 50 million chickens are slaughtered for food in Canada, 600 million in the United Kingdom, and 6 billion in the United States—about 2 chickens per person in Canada, 10 per person in the United Kingdom, and 24 per person in the United States. Chickens raised for meat live in appalling conditions. Little regard is given to the birds' physical capacity to feel pain. Slaughter practices are so sloppy and rushed that the death of many chickens is unnecessarily long and painful.

A chicken raised for meat begins life inside a breeding farm incubator. After a few days, the chick is nail-clipped, de-beaked, vaccinated, and moved to an indoor growth building (or broiler shed) at a factory farm.

Broiler chickens, unlike egg-laying hens, are not kept in battery cages but are left loose in growth houses to keep their flesh free of the bruises and blisters caused by rubbing against the sides of wire cages. Living conditions in growth houses are not much better, however. The chickens spend their entire lives in overcrowded conditions. From 10,000 to 75,000 birds are kept in one growth building. By slaughter time, when the birds have grown, the crowding in the buildings is so severe that it is estimated that each bird has as little as 0.65 square foot (0.06 square metre) of space.[7]

As the goal is to develop the biggest birds in the shortest possible time, the environment inside the building is controlled to trick the birds into believing that it is day when the lights are on and night when they are off. The chickens eat during the hour-long simulated day and sleep in the artificial darkness. This practice keeps the birds calmer and makes them less active, so they gain weight faster.

The basic low-cost diet of factory-farm chickens consists of unsaleable poultry parts combined with hormones, antibiotics, and additives such as xanthophyll, which increases the yellow color of the chicken's skin to make it more appealing to shoppers. Some chickens are given chicken manure mixed with feed to keep feeding costs even lower.[8]

The natural life span of a broiler chicken is about seven years. On an intensive factory farm, it is about nine weeks. Factory-farm producers refer to the chickens as a crop that they harvest about five times a year.[9]

The growth buildings are cleaned only after each crop of broilers has been sent to market. The birds spend their entire lives standing or squatting on piles of their own droppings, which have become hard-packed from their weight. Drugs are routinely given to prevent outbreaks of disease and the spread of bacterial contamination from the manure. Many broilers suffer from constant diarrhea. When this type of manure hardens, many animals develop ulcerated feet and hock burns from walking on it.

Ventilation in the growth buildings is very poor. During summer months, many broilers suffer overheating, strokes, dehydration, heart attacks, and respiratory diseases due to excessive dust. In winter, ventilation is often reduced even more, and the animals' manure becomes damp and emits an overpowering stench of ammonia, which contributes to respiratory illnesses.

Like the slaughter of all other food animals, the slaughter of chickens is done mechanically and callously, with little or no regard for the animals' suffering. Workers usually storm the growth buildings during the night when the birds are asleep. Hysteria and panic ensue. The workers grab the chickens by the legs and wings and stuff them into slatted plastic crates for transportation to the slaughterhouse (in North America, sometimes located hundreds of miles away). Two or three chickens are packed into a 2-by-3-foot (0.5-by-1-m) crate. Fragile bones are broken and joints dislocated by the rough handling. If the transport truck arrives at the slaughtering plant near closing time, the chickens are not killed until the next morning and are left in the plastic crates all night without food or water.

Until the time of transport, the chickens live away from bright sunlight and extremes in weather. Their first encounter with the elements is shocking. Millions of chickens die every year from shock, heat stress, extreme cold, exhaustion, or suffocation on the way to slaughter.[10]

At slaughtering plants, the chickens are roughly removed from their crates, shackled by their legs, hung upside down on a moving conveyor belt, and electronically stunned. Stunning is supposed to render the chickens unconscious, but with low-voltage stunning (70 volts), only about 40 percent of the birds are properly stunned by the time their throats are cut.[11] Thus, many chickens are fully conscious and capable of feeling extreme pain and terror during the entire procedure. Throat cutting causes suffering when the automatic revolving blade is not manually adjusted to the size of the bird. The chickens' feathers are removed by scalding. Some chickens are still alive when they enter the scalding stage.[12]

The Life of Turkeys

Turkeys, a close relative of the pheasant and the partridge, are wild in nature and terribly ill-suited to captivity. In many parts of North America, turkeys still live and breed in the wild. The captivity and breeding of turkeys on factory farms is fairly recent. Before 1965, turkeys were raised on farms in relatively small numbers for the Thanksgiving and Christmas markets. They are now raised in over-crowded conditions in massive growth housing systems.

On their fifth day of life, 70 to 80 percent of all turkeys are de-beaked. Male birds kept for breeding are de-beaked a second time when sixteen weeks old. Errors and carelessness often lead to permanent injuries.[13] In overcrowded conditions, failure to de-beak can lead to severe injuries and high mortality from self-mutilation and cannibalism. The crowding is so intense and stress levels so high on factory farms that even de-beaked turkeys relentlessly peck each other's feathers and eyes.[14]

As many as 15,000 turkeys are kept in one growth building, where they are subjected to the same overcrowding and unsanitary conditions as broiler chickens. The buildings are kept semi-dark in an attempt to control aggression and cannibalism, but this practice has proven to be of little use. Every year, 7 percent of the young birds (approx-imately four weeks old) die as a result of the crowding typical of intensive rearing systems. Included in this figure are the many young turkeys that never learn to find their feed or water and simply starve to death. Also included are the weak and ill turkeys that are trampled on and injured by stronger birds and go unnoticed among the large number of turkeys. Growth buildings are cleaned only after each crop of turkeys has been reared and sent to slaughter. Under these conditions, sick and injured birds are not noticed by the producers until the entire batch is sent to market and the grounds are cleaned.

The large accumulation of droppings and the lack of fresh air and sunshine cause much illness. Turkeys confined in the overcrowded growth buildings stand on wet and crusty piles of excrement. Many develop painful ulcerated foot pads and eventually become partially or totally lame. In an attempt to control the spread of disease, turkeys are routinely given antibiotics.

Because the turkey market demands big, meaty birds, turkeys have become victims of genetic manipulation. Their bodies have been restructured through selective breeding to grow to a size and weight too great for the strength of their legs. The result is birds with weak, malformed bone structures and in some cases crippled, deformed legs.

Reproduction must be accomplished through artificial insemination because natural fertilization cannot take place. The turkeys are not alive long enough to go through their natural breeding cycles, and their heavy weight and weak bones make them incapable of mating naturally.[15] Male birds selected specifically for the purpose of breeding are milked for semen every two to three days. Doses of collected semen are forced into the vaginas of selected hens.[16] Both male and female birds suffer stress from the handling involved. Once the males have passed their semen-producing prime (at about one year) and the females their egg-laying peak (also at about one year), they are slaughtered.

The average life span of a turkey is approximately ten years. Factory-farm turkeys are slaughtered when they are between twelve and sixteen weeks old. Before slaughter, turkeys are deprived of food for twelve hours or more. The centerpiece of bountiful holiday feasts thus goes to its death starved of food.[17] For transportation to slaughter, the turkeys are caught and stuffed into bins. Rough handling of the frightened birds causes extreme stress and fear. At the slaughterhouse, the turkeys are shackled by their feet, hoisted into the air, and moved by conveyor belt to where they are electronically stunned. The time on the conveyor belt, which can be up to six minutes, inflicts additional suffering, particularly on birds with antotrochanteric degeneration, a painful hip joint condition that causes lameness in almost 80 percent of male breeding birds.[18] Turkeys are generally stunned by a hand device. While being held upside down, many of the birds arch their necks and thus miss the full impact of the stunning. These unfortunate birds then go through the rest of the slaughtering procedure, including the cutting of their throats, while still semi-conscious.

Although used as a symbol in Christmas and Thanksgiving rituals, factory-farm turkeys have little to be thankful for in their short, harsh lives.

Cows as Sources of Dairy Products, Veal, and Beef

Cows are gentle, peaceful animals, content to graze slowly across a field and to stand or lie down for hours chewing their cud. They live naturally in herds in which each cow has a place in the social hierarchy and lives in harmony with the others.[19]

In factory-farm conditions, dairy cows, veal calves, and beef cattle are raised without consideration for their instincts or needs. Their lives are structured to produce the highest possible return, with little regard for their health or well-being.

In North America, cows are branded on the face for identification, without anesthetic or analgesic. The 3-inch (7-cm) mark is burned on the side of the cow's face, just below the eye. Another painful procedure is dehorning, which is believed to reduce injuries among animals and farm-hands in crowded pens. Dehorning is commonly done by melting down or gouging out the horns. In the melt-down method, a device similar to a high-temperature soldering unit is put directly on the horns and held in place for ten seconds; the heat melts the horns. In the gouging method, a tool is used to gouge out the horns of calves under the age of three months. Gouging usually pulls out about half an inch of the skin surrounding the horns and thus subjects the calf to bleeding and trauma.

Dairy Cows and Their Lives of Continual Pregnancies

Female cows have strong maternal instincts. They are conscientious and attentive mothers and form strong bonds with their newborn calves. William Dempster Hoard, a nineteenth-century journalist and dairy industry crusader, posted this notice in his own barn: "Remember that this is the home of Mothers. Treat each cow as a Mother should be treated."[20] On factory farms, dairy cows are not treated as mothers should be. *New Scientist Magazine* describes the dairy cow as "leading one hell of a life. Each year she hopefully produces a calf, which means that for nine months of the year she is pregnant. And for nine months of each year she is milked twice a day. For six months she is both pregnant and lactating."[21] Dairy cows are treated as calf- and milk-producing machines.

When barely out of the calf stage, dairy cows on factory farms are started on a continuous cycle of pregnancies. At eighteen to twenty-four months of age, the cows are artificially inseminated, a practice done once a year for the rest of their calf-producing lives. Cows labelled super producers of top stock calves are further used by having their embryos surgically removed each time they are impregnated. They can then be inseminated again to keep producing top stock embryos. The embryos taken from these cows are implanted into "inferior" cows that carry the implanted embryos to term.

Following the birth of her calf, the cow produces colostrum, a yellowish milk rich in protein, nutrients, and antibodies. Colostrum is the main form of nutrition for the newborn calf. The calf is allowed to remain with the mother and feed on colostrum to ensure that it will survive the first few critical days of life. A few days later, when the mother starts producing regular milk, the newborn calf is taken away to prevent its consuming milk intended for sale to human consumers. The separation of mother and calf inflicts "anguish on both. Cows are highly intelligent, and attachment between the calf and the mother is particularly strong."[22]

After being taken from their mothers, newborn calves are reared in two groups. Females are raised as dairy cows and are housed in free stall or tie stall barns; male calves are either raised on the same premises or sent away to be raised as veal calves.

In free stall barns, cows are kept in a holding pen where they have some freedom of movement. Twice daily they are walked to a milking room, milked by an automated system, and returned to the pen. In more intensive systems, the cows live in narrow, cage-like cubicles known as tie stalls. Each stall is approximately 7 feet long and 5 to 8 feet wide (2.5 m by 2 m). Cows living in these stalls are completely confined. They are kept in place by a rope tied to the neck; other than a few steps forward or backward, they are unable to walk or turn around and can lie down only in discomfort. Milking machines are brought to the individual stalls, so the cows do not even walk to the milking room.

In both systems, straw for lying on is not provided. Floors are made of wood, packed earth, or slatted concrete, all of which become muddy and slippery from the animals' excrement. Standing and lying on hard floors causes skin irritations, infections, lameness, joint disorders, and mastitis, a painful inflammation of the udder, believed to affect one-third of all dairy cows.[23]

Dairy cows are not allowed out to graze in pastures. Their diet consists of high-protein concentrated feeds developed to increase milk production and keep it at abnormally high levels. Concentrated feeds are associated with many metabolic disorders. In one painful condition called ketosis, the cow breaks down her own body stores to produce more milk. Untreated, ketosis often leads to severe weight loss and infertility. Laminitis, a painful inflammation of the hoof, aggravated by standing on concrete or soiled hard floors for a long time, is also linked to high-energy feeds.

Under normal living conditions, with the right food and exercise, dairy cows live fifteen or twenty years. In the intensive systems of factory farming, dairy cows live on average three to five years. When physically depleted from the continuous cycle of calf and milk production and no longer productive, the cows are slaughtered. Dairy cows provide an estimated 80 percent of the ground beef used in the fast food industry.[24]

The Veal Calf: From Birth to Slaughter in Sixteen Weeks

The most unfortunate calves are the 1.5 million calves raised annually for white veal in North America.

Many veal calves do not see daylight until they are on the way to slaughter. The lifespan of calves raised for white veal is just a few months, and the quality of their lives is abysmal. The calves are denied the most basic physical and psychological necessities. Living conditions for white veal calves in many intensive systems are at best stressful and can be terrifying. Separated from its mother when just a few days old, the calf is transported to an auction market, where it is bought by a veal producer. In many cases, the calf has not had enough time to nurse fully on colostrum and so has not built up resistance to disease.[25]

On North American veal farms, the calves are housed in what the industry calls veal crates. Rows of dozens or hundreds of these crates fill a factory-farm building. Each cage-like cubicle, with bars on the sides, measures on average between 24 and 28 inches in width and 60 inches in length (60 cm by 150 cm). The calf is only slightly smaller than these dimensions. Some crates have been known to measure as little as 22 inches in width and 54 inches in length (56 cm by 137 cm). This crate is where the calf spends its entire sixteen weeks of life.

The calf is roped or chained at the neck so that it is unable to move its head more than a few inches from side to side. It is also unable to turn around, to groom itself, or to lie down and fully stretch its legs. All movement is discouraged to prevent muscle development, which would give the meat a tougher texture.

Calves are naturally active and playful animals;[26] the lack of social interaction and exercise contributes to high levels of stress, anxiety, and restlessness. The industry refuses to acknowledge that this type of restriction is cruel. However, in an attempt to reduce stress and restlessness, many producers keep temperatures high and the buildings in permanent semi-darkness.

For quick removal of waste, the floor of the crates is slatted to allow the waste to fall through and collect in a holding pan on the floor below. Slatted floors are not suited to hoofed animals, and many calves suffer painful swelling of the knee joints and extreme discomfort of the feet.[27]

Because the calves are not given solid food, many suffer from chronic diarrhea and must live in an area that is continuously soiled. The constant presence of watery waste attracts flies and other insects that plague the calf. The restricted calf's inability to move enough to scratch itself further contributes to an already high level of stress and anxiety.[28] It is not uncommon for one out of ten calves living in such conditions to die before reaching the age of three months, a figure considered acceptable by producers.

Veal calves are fed an unnatural diet to ensure that their flesh stays as pale as possible.[29] They are deprived of all solid food and fed only a liquid formula consisting of powdered milk, high levels of fat-promoting additives, sugar, vitamins, and drugs such as penicillin.

Temperatures in the barn are kept high to make the calves thirsty, and water is withheld so the calves will drink the formula, which, combined with the calves' restricted movement, causes quick weight gain.

If the newborn calves were allowed to drink their mothers' milk, the milk would provide enough nutrients to sustain the calves, and additives and vitamins would not be required. Under natural conditions, the nursing calves would also begin eating grass at about two weeks of age and thus obtain iron and required vitamins. On factory farms, the calves' intake of iron and vitamin B12 is restricted to its absolute lowest; the immediate requirement is met, but there is no surplus to be stored. The calves are kept chronically anemic.[30] Straw bedding is not provided, because straw is a source of iron. The calves would eat the straw, and their flesh would become darker. In a desperate attempt to obtain iron, the calves resort to licking their own urine, which contains small amounts of iron. They also lick the metal fittings of the crates. Preventing these practices is another justification the industry gives for restricting the calves' movement.

The calves suffer from lack of contact with their mothers and denial of their urge to suck. They engage in repetitive, neurotic behavior such as rolling their tongues and licking, sucking, and eating the wood of the crates.

After fourteen to sixteen weeks of miserable existence, the veal calves, suffering from maternal deprivation and anemia and in some cases also from stomach ulcers, abscesses, anemia, and lameness are taken from their crates. On shaky legs, they are forced into trucks and transported to slaughter.

Beef Cattle

Calves raised to be beef cattle are allowed to remain with their mothers until weaning is complete. Once weaned, the calves are raised for market on the premises or taken to auction and sold to operators elsewhere.[31] The time needed to turn a calf into saleable beef used to be three years. On factory farms, it is fourteen months.[32]

The young male calves are castrated. A veterinarian is required to perform the surgery on calves older than two months, using anesthetics and pain-relieving drugs. However, castration may be carried out on calves under two months by a non-medical person and without the use of an anesthetic. Thus, to save on expenses, most producers castrate calves before they are two months old. Hemorrhages, infections, tetanus, and maggot infestations are a few of the possible complications.[33]

Factory-farm beef calves are raised and housed in either indoor or outdoor feed lots. Although these systems house the animals in conditions that allow some freedom of movement, neither provide humane living conditions. Indoor feedlots house hundreds of calves in pens. The large factory-like buildings provide shelter but little else. Some are not equipped with adequate air cooling and ventilation systems. As a result, during the summer months, the stench from excrement is overwhelming. Strong disinfectants, germicides, and bacteria-killing sprays are used to control the flies and pests attracted to the manure. The hard slatted floors and absence of straw in the pens can lead to partial or total lameness in animals whose hooves and legs are not designed for standing on hard floors.

Most beef calves are housed in the open air. In midwestern areas of Canada and the United States, outdoor lots contain tens of thousands of calves destined for the beef market. These lots are vast pens or fields sectioned by concrete ducts that hold feed and carry water to the animals being fattened for slaughter. During dry summer months, the ground turns into hard, packed soil covered with droppings. Both the stench of accumulated excrement and the degree of dust are extreme. In winter, when the fields turn into cold mud and slush, the animals cannot lie down to rest for even short periods. The animals that lie down under these conditions do so only because they are ill or suffering from extreme fatigue.

Beef calves are fed mainly legumes, soy beans, corn (maize), barley and other grains, protein supplements, and growth-promoting drugs. This highly concentrated diet, combined with lack of exercise, leads to quick weight gain. But cattle are ruminant (cud-chewing) animals whose systems are designed to digest grasses. Diets high in grain cause damage to the digestive system and frustrate the cattle's natural urge to ruminate. In an attempt to obtain roughage and satisfy the ruminant urge, some cattle constantly lick their own coats and the coats of other calves. Fur then accumulates in the digestive system, causing ulcers and abscesses.[34] This painful condition is detected only after the calf has been slaughtered.

Like other cows, beef cattle living in such unnatural conditions suffer high levels of stress, which makes them susceptible to disease. Producers then give them antibiotics and sulfa drugs to control possible epidemics.

After a life of fourteen months (compared to a natural life span of fifteen to twenty years), beef calves are loaded onto trucks and driven to slaughterhouses.

Pigs As Pork

"Forget the pig is an animal. Treat him like a machine in a factory. Schedule treatment like you would lubrication. Breeding like the first step in an assembly line. And marketing like the delivery of finished stock."

- J. Brynes, Hog Farm Management

Pigs are intelligent, sociable animals, with the same capacity for learning that dogs have. They can be kept as pets, house-trained, and taught to obey commands. Pigs show a natural curiosity when they are in an interesting environment, and they love to explore new places. In groups, they establish a social order and a system of interacting with each other. Pigs enjoy rooting (digging up the ground with their snouts) and wallowing (rolling around in mud to cool off and keep insects away).

Sows have a strong maternal instinct and form close and lasting bonds with their young. The piglets are naturally playful. "When we give them [the piglets] fresh straw," says free-range farmer Mark Peterson, "they love to run around in it and play, and occasionally you'd see a 500-pound sow running around the pen chasing after and playing tag with her little pigs."[35]

Pigs on modern factory farms are not allowed to do their natural activities.[36] They are confined in cages barely larger than their own bodies and have no physical or social contact with other pigs.

The Life of a Breeding Sow

Many male pigs on factory farms lose their instinct for reproduction, and many females develop irregular menstruation cycles. Producers regulate reproduction by giving hormones and using artificial insemination.

Top-stock quality sows are impregnated four times per year. Once pregnant, a sow is moved into a gestation building, where she is kept either in a small pen with other pregnant sows or in solitary confinement in an individual pen. The individual pen is only large enough for the sow to stand up and lie down; she cannot turn around or walk. According to producers, this restriction saves space, makes feeding and inspection easier, and avoids doing time-consuming examinations of individual sows housed in groups. Individual pens are to be phased out in the U.K. by 1998.

Pigs confined in box stalls often develop behavioral disorders. They habitually bite the bars of the stall, chew with empty mouths, and repetitively rub the bridge of their nose on the cage bars. The habit of "mourning," or sitting for long periods of time with their heads hanging low and eyes shut, is also found in pigs housed in solitary confinement. Sitting is an unnatural and awkward position for a pig and is usually just a transitory movement between lying down and standing up. Pigs in groups sit for only a few minutes, but in solitary confinement pigs may sit in the mourning position for many hours.[37]

Another form of restriction for sows is tethering. The sow is tied up in a cagelike cubicle. A rope or chain tied around the sow's neck or middle and secured to the ground impedes almost all movement. Tethering is done to lower food costs by keeping the sows from moving about and burning calories. The following is an account of the reaction of sows being tethered for the first time: "Following a brief and gentle tug on the tether chain, the sows threw themselves violently backwards, straining against the tether. . . . Sows thrashed their heads about as they twisted and turned in their struggle to free themselves. Often loud screams were emitted and occasionally individuals crashed bodily against the side bars of the tether stall. This sometimes resulted in the sows collapsing to the floors."[38]

Once the piglets are born, the only interaction allowed between mother and babies is suckling between the bars of the stall. The piglets are weaned much earlier than normal and then taken away from their mother, to her distress. As soon as she is physically able, the sow is impregnated again, and the cycle of restriction and confinement continues. As long as the sow is able to become pregnant and the stock she produces is acceptable, she will not be slaughtered.

Some people argue that because these sows are specifically bred for confinement, no cruelty is involved. However, when a factory-farm sow is taken out of the intensive system and placed on a free-range open-air farm, she immediately begins to build a nest for the litter she is expecting, even though she never before had the opportunity to build one.[39] A factory-farm sow giving birth on a straw-lined bed for the first time continuously pulls straw toward the piglets she is bearing. She knows instinctively that the newborns need to be as warm and as comfortable as possible.[40] Sows giving birth in factory farms paw at the ground trying to make a nest even when there is nothing there for them to use.

The Treatment of Piglets

Piglets are born with very sharp teeth. Their teeth are clipped to prevent the piglets injuring themselves or other piglets. Their tails are also docked (cut off) and their ears notched for identification. When the male piglets are a few days old, they are castrated. The industry believes that pigs whose testicles have been surgically removed make better food animals. All of these procedures are done without anesthetic or analgesic. The piglets are force-weaned at three or four weeks of age. Pigs' natural weaning age is about the twelfth week.[41] Producers are attempting to further reduce costs by shortening the weaning period even more. Research is now under way to develop a pig that could be taken from its mother a few days after birth and confined in a cage where automated feeding systems would replace the mother, so that sows could be forced to give birth five times a year instead of four.[42]

Once the piglets are weaned, they are moved into a growth building, where they spend the next eight weeks. In the growth building, two or three animals are housed in each flat-deck cage. The cages are stacked two tiers high. Flat-deck cages have no straw or any other type of bedding. The floor either is of sloping concrete so that droppings accumulate at the lowest point or has slats to allow waste to fall through and collect in a holding pan below. Pigs, which have a highly developed sense of smell, are confronted day and night by the stench of the collected urine and feces. Piglets housed on the lower tier are subjected to splatters of waste falling from the cages above. Like other hoofed animals, pigs suffer from being forced to stand on hard surfaces. Many pigs in factory farms have painfully splayed legs, arthritis, and lameness. Many young pigs that have been prematurely separated from their mothers and confined in small cages develop behavioral disorders such as flank nuzzling, tail biting, and navel sucking. In an attempt to reduce the stress that causes these disorders, some producers keep the growth buildings in permanent semi-darkness.[43]

When the pigs are eight weeks old, they are moved to a "finishing" building where they will spend their final four months of life. There, the pigs are unconfined but are subjected to extremely crowded conditions. The temperature is kept high to discourage movement and promote weight gain. When the pigs reach the desired market weight, at six or seven months of age, they are sent to the slaughterhouse.

The Unhappy Ending: Slaughter

"From an early age, I have abjured the use of meat, and the time will come when men will look upon the murder of animals as they look upon the murder of men."
- *Leonardo da Vinci*

When animals arrive at a slaughterhouse, they are put in holding pens. From the pen, they walk in single file down an alley where a V-shaped conveyor-restrainer system closes in on the animal's body and carries it down the line to the stunning quarters. The U.K. organization Compassion in World Farming estimates that a large percentage of food animals are not properly stunned before being slaughtered. Part of the problem is attributed to poorly maintained equipment and the rest to a lack of concern about humane treatment.

A number of methods are used to stun food animals. The captive bolt pistol and electric current are the most common. Large animals such as cows and large calves are stunned with the captive bolt pistol. The captive bolt pistol is propelled by a blank cartridge or compressed air. It is fired through the skull, penetrates the brain, and causes instant unconsciousness. Done correctly, captive bolt stunning is the best available method of rendering an animal unconscious. But if the animal moves its head sideways at the moment of firing, the result is a "blotched," or blemished, shot, which is painful for the animal. Electric stunning is done with a hand-held device that sends an electric current through the animal's brain to produce instant unconsciousness.[44] If the current fails to pass through the brain properly, the animal is paralyzed but stays fully conscious and is able to feel pain.[45] In order to work properly, the electric tongs must be held in place on the animal's head for at least seven seconds. In poorly operated slaughterhouses, tongs are rarely applied for the correct length of time because of carelessness and rushing, causing yet more pain and suffering.[46]

Immediately after the animal is rendered unconscious, one of its hind legs is fastened to a hoist chain, and its body is lifted into the air. The animal's head is positioned directly over a large concrete pit, and the slaughterer slashes the throat. Blood pours forth and collects in the concrete pit. In a short time, the animal bleeds to death.

At many slaughterhouses, cruel treatment ranges from lack of compassion toward panic-stricken animals to deliberate acts of aggression. Sickening reports of animal abuse are still made about day-to-day operations.

Richard Koury, senior inspector with the Ontario Humane Society in Newmarket, Ontario, has been inspecting slaughterhouses for more than a decade. He says the following about slaughter practices: "I've seen chicken, pig, beef, and geese slaughter. We can't be there every day, so it is very difficult to say whether every animal is killed humanely. [The slaughterers] aren't paid great salaries. And you have to ask yourself, what kind of person can kill animals eight hours a day, five days a week? They still use the cane [to hit the animals]. In some cases, they use a large piece of rubber, that is snapped across an uncooperative [frightened] animal's back . . . it makes a loud noise but doesn't hurt the meat. The electric prods are used, and you do get the occasional sadist who wants to stick it up between a cow's legs and watch her jump."[47]

In an article in the *Washington Star*, Temple Grandin reported witnessing the following incident: "One day I walked around the corner of a plant and caught a person in the act of ramming an electric prod twelve inches long down a steer's throat because the animal refused to enter a stunning pen. The animal was lying on the floor of the lead-up chute and the man just kept shoving the prod deeper down its throat."[48] At another plant, a man in charge of stunning animals was taking "sadistic delight in shooting both the animal's eyes out with a stunner [gun] before killing it. He thought it was funny, and would jump up and down and laugh."[49]

Too few inspectors or too few concerned inspectors present during loading, off-loading, pre-slaughter, and slaughter accounts for numerous other abuses and mistreatment of the animals at the hands of unconcerned workers. Some of these workers are notorious for being rough and lacking compassion when dealing with frightened or injured animals. One compelling argument for vegetarianism is that the brutalizing work in a slaughterhouse is something no human being should be expected to perform.

In the assembly-line approach to animal slaughter, ill or crippled animals unable to walk on their own are rarely helped or given extra consideration. Instead, they are left in the transport truck and are trampled on by healthier animals. Some are pushed, kicked, prodded, or dragged to slaughter,[50] even though the Humane Slaughter Act in the U.S. and the Cruelty to Animals Criminal Code in Canada forbid the dragging of injured animals. Dragging is legally permitted only after the animal has been properly stunned and made insensitive to pain.

An example of this kind of abuse was recorded in an article in the Toronto Sun by a newspaper reporter who posed as an animal husbandry (agriculture) student to gain access to a stockyard. During the unloading of the animals, "pigs were kicked, pulled, and pushed into overcrowded pens, while workers swore and beat them with wooden canes, whips, or 72-volt electric prods." The article went on to describe how "one pig stood alone in a pen, trembling and soaked in blood. Its legs were bent awkwardly and it was trying to edge slowly towards an empty water trough . . .workers were seen forcing such pigs, which they call 'spreaders,' up ramps using electric prods."[51]

When confronted with horror stories like this, the slaughter industry argues that these incidents are rare. People in the animal welfare movement, however, believe that such episodes have only rarely been *witnessed*. Compassion for individual animals is not a high priority in slaughterhouses. Turning helpless beings into undamaged carcasses as quickly and cost-effectively as possible is the highest priority.

Religious Slaughter Practices Affect Every Meat-Eater

"If the Jewish people knew what was going on, they would insist that the Case-Javits amendment [which exempts kosher slaughter from the prohibition on shackling and hoisting conscious animals] be replaced."
- *Max Schnapp, Founder of the Jewish Committee for Humane Slaughter*

Federal laws in the United States regulating slaughter practices have had the unintended and unfortunate consequence of turning previously humane religious slaughter into cruel slaughter. Since a large percentage of kosher meat sold in Canada comes from the United States, the practices there affect both countries. And not only buyers of kosher meat are affected, since some meat from religious slaughterhouses is not labelled as such.

In ancient times, it was realized that eating the meat of animals found "still," or dead, caused disease and illness. Jewish elders forbade the consumption of meat that came from animals that did not move at the time of slaughter. Thus began the ritual practice of ensuring that an animal was alive and able to move at the time it was killed for human consumption. Today, a small number of North American Orthodox Jews still follow the tradition of eating only kosher, or clean, meat.

The ancient Hebrews, who were concerned about animal welfare, stipulated that the killing was to be done as quickly and humanely as possible, in keeping with the Talmudic exhortation that Jews must have reverence for all life. In the Jewish slaughter ritual, the killing is done by a trained slaughterer using a flawlessly sharp knife. The killing is done as quickly and as carefully as possible, without unnecessary pain or suffering for the animal.

This method of producing kosher meat was practiced in the United States until 1906, when the Pure Food and Drug Act stipulated that a slaughtered animal could not, for hygiene reasons, fall into the blood of a previously killed animal. This regulation did not do much to improve hygenic practices in slaughterhouses, but it resulted in the practice of chaining the animals and lifting them off the floor by one hind leg while they were still fully conscious.[52]

Seventy-two years later, it was finally acknowledged that shackling and hoisting a fully conscious animal caused pain and suffering. In 1978, the U.S. Congress passed the Humane Slaughter Act, which specifies that animals must be rendered unconscious before being shackled and hoisted. As Jewish ritual slaughter requires that animals be conscious and unblemished before being slain, kosher slaughtering was exempted from the Humane Slaughter Act.[53]

The law requiring hoisting combined with the exemption from stunning transformed ritual slaughter into the cruel and complicated act it has become today. It is estimated that since 1978 between one and two million cattle and about one million calves, sheep, and lambs have gone to their death in religious slaughter every year, many of them terrified and fully aware of what is taking place around them.[54]

Killing Practices

The animal's neck must be outstretched so that the four major blood vessels and the windpipe can be severed in one quick cut. This technique allows the maximum amount of blood to flow from the animal's body to cause almost instant unconsciousness. In many plants in North America, a clamp is placed in the suspended animal's nostril, and the neck is outstretched by a powerful air cylinder which may apply as much as 400 pounds of pull to facilitate the slashing of the throat.[55] But even with the painful outstretching of the animal's neck, a quick death depends on the skillfulness of the slaughterer. If he is able to cause immediate collapse of the animal, there is little suffering for the animal. However, if he is inexperienced or less skillful and does not sever all four major blood vessels at the same time, the animal is subjected to a slow and painful death.

When done correctly, the religious slaughter of animals is no more crude or violent than other kinds of slaughter. But of greater concern in religious slaughter is the shackling and hoisting of the animals while they are still alive and fully conscious, without benefit of stunning. Shackling and hoisting tears flesh and ligaments, breaks bones, and ruptures joints around the hip and knee area. Depending on the efficiency of the slaughterhouse, the animals spend two to five minutes suspended by one hind leg while being conveyed, bellowing and violently jerking, to slaughter. Delays along the slaughter line mean a longer time in this agonizing position.[56]

Of the hundreds of thousands of calves and lambs killed annually for kosher meat, nearly all are fully conscious at the time of shackling and hoisting. Only a small percentage of large cattle are shackled and hoisted, but it is a large absolute number of cattle that are subjected to this suffering.

When the animal reaches the slaughter section, its throat is slashed, and there is an immediate outpouring of blood. Orthodox Jews are not to consume meat from an animal whose blood has not been fully drained. Realistically, to assure complete draining, either a liquid would have to be pumped into the veins and arteries of the carcass or the veins would have to be removed. Since the veins in the hindquarters are small and numerous and their removal would be time-consuming and extremely expensive, the poorly drained hind portions that do not qualify as kosher may be sold in stores in North America as regular meat.[57] People who buy non-kosher meat may thus unknowingly buy the meat of animals that were not stunned and were fully conscious at the time of slaughter.[58]

The Introduction of Humane Reforms

Because of pressure from animal advocacy groups and the concern of a small number of people in the slaughter industry, "humane" slaughter equipment has been introduced. One example is the ASPCA (American Society for the Prevention of Cruelty to Animals) pen, which was introduced in 1964. It is a narrow stall with an opening in front for the animal's head. A lift under the animal's body prevents the animal from collapsing while a chin lift raises its head and holds it in place for the slaughterer. After the animal's throat has been cut, a shackle is put around one back leg and the animal is hoisted out through the side.[59]

Such relatively humane restraining pens are used in about 60 per cent of ritual slaughter in the United States today; 40 percent of ritually slaughtered animals are hung upside down while still conscious. The practice of hoisting conscious animals is still legal in the United States. England and Canada prohibit it.

While attempts to make slaughtering methods more humane are commendable, the slaughtering of animals for food necessarily causes suffering. This suffering is, of course, completely unnecessary, because humans can live healthily without eating meat.

CHAPTER 4

Vegetarianism for a Healthier Environment

"Vegetarianism creates both healthier people
and a healthier planet."
- *People for the Ethical Treatment of Animals,
Washington, D.C.*

A vegetarian diet causes a minuscule amount of environmental destruction and pollution compared to the amount caused by a diet that includes animal products. Over the course of the average meat eater's life, he or she consumes approximately fifty cows, calves, and pigs in total, more than a thousand chickens and turkeys, and thousands of fish.[1] Besides causing the miserable existence and slaughter of animals and endangering the meat eater's own health, meat consumption also endangers the planet. Raising animals is an extremely inefficient way of producing food for humans. The existence of enormous numbers of farm animals contributes significantly to the pollution of air, water, and soil, depletes natural resources, and causes massive destruction of forests and grasslands.

Inefficient Use of Land

More than 80 percent of North America's rich, harvestable land is currently used to grow crops, but only a small fraction of the harvest of these crops is for human consumption. Most of it is used to feed animals. Raising feed for animals on rich soil is a tremendous waste of agricultural land and resources.

As Frances Moore Lappé points out, "An acre of cereals can produce *five times* more protein than an acre devoted to meat production; legumes (beans, peas, lentils) can produce *ten times* more; and leafy vegetables *fifteen times* more."[2] Soy beans, for example, are a nutritious food for humans, whether eaten as beans, tofu, or tempeh or fermented into soy sauce or miso. Ken McMullen of the Canadian Organic Growers states that Canada "could easily grow enough soy beans to feed one-third to one-half of the world's population in plant protein. We have a tremendous abundance of agricultural land, if we would only work with it properly." Instead, almost all the soy beans grown in Canada are fed to chickens and pigs. In northern Ontario and Quebec, farms that could grow soy beans instead produce barley for livestock feed.[3]

Pollution of Water and Soil

More than 80 percent of North America's water consumption is used for the production of food animals.[4] In addition, the production of meat is responsible for most of North America's water pollution—more than other industry and households combined.[5] Beef-fattening farms, for example, discharge massive amounts of phosphates, nitrates, and fats into waterways. Dung from factory farms drains into slurry pits, many of which leak into waterways, causing further water pollution. Slaughterhouses are major polluters of rivers and streams, filling them with poisonous residues of animal waste.

Michael Schwab of Canadian Vegans for Animal Rights says: "What people don't understand is that stopping cruelty towards animals is going to make life better for people, because the cruelty is causing terrible pollution. The crowding of [poultry] birds, for example, is leading to more antibiotics and pesticides being used to kill infestations. These in turn pollute our water table."[6]

In addition, factory farming is a serious source of topsoil pollution. A typical factory egg-laying building, holding approximately 60,000 hens, produces more than 80 tons of manure per week. An average-sized pork farm creates more than 27 tons of manure and 32 tons of urine weekly.[7] In "A Report on Intensive Livestock: A Canadian Review, Interim Report," Jim Haskill of Environment Canada cited the following waste management problems: insufficient storage, run-off pollution from manure stacks, and problems with odor and raw untreated manure applied directly on cropland.

With all of these problems combined, it is estimated that up to a third of the world's cropland will be destroyed in the next twenty years if the present rate of top-soil damage continues.

Destruction of Forests

Trees, the living lungs of the earth, increase the earth's oxygen supply and absorb carbon dioxide and other environmental pollutants. They absorb water, evaporate it through their leaves, and send it back into the atmosphere. By destroying large numbers of trees to clear land for crops to feed animals, we are leaving future generations a legacy of increased pollution, higher carbon dioxide levels in the atmosphere, and food shortages.

Approximately 50 acres (20 ha) of trees are cut down every minute: 28 million acres (11 million ha) of land are cleared annually for crops and fuel. The rapid and irreversible destruction of the Central and South American rain forests is continuing at an alarming rate. Whole villages of people are being forced from their ancestral lands, where they have acted as stewards of the rainforests. Animal habitats and plants used for medicines are being destroyed along with the trees.[8] Continued meat consumption causes continued destruction of the environment upon which the survival of our species and every other species on the planet depends.

World Hunger

While 800 million people face starvation around the world,[9] people of richer nations are wasting land, water, and crops in order to eat meat.[10] Although world hunger will not end until there are major political and economic changes worldwide, a large-scale change to vegetarianism would certainly alleviate demands on the use of land and cause less waste of natural resources.

CHAPTER 5

Writing Letters to Encourage Change

"All that is needed for the triumph of evil
is for good men to do nothing."
- *Edmund Burke*

"Consumer awareness and consumer pressure
are the most effective means we have
in eliminating the health hazards posed by factory farming
and ending needless animal suffering."
- *Humane Farming Association,*
San Francisco, California

Writing to the Government

I encourage you to write to your elected representatives and the appropriate senior government officials to ask them to implement ongoing programs to promote vegetarianism and educate the general public, especially schoolchildren, about the advantages of a vegetarian diet—for human health, for animals, and for the environment—and about how to make sure a vegetarian diet is well balanced.

In Canada, write to:

Minister of Health
House of Commons
Ottawa, Ontario K1A 0A6

Minister of Agriculture
House of Commons
Ottawa, Ontario K1A 0A6

Minister of the Environment
House of Commons
Ottawa, Ontario K1A 0A6

Contact any school or library for the names and addresses of your provincial Minister of Education and local school board members.

In the United States, write to:

Secretary of Health and Human Services
Department of Health and Human Services
200 Independence Avenue SW
Washington, DC 20201

Secretary of Agriculture
Department of Agriculture
14th Street and Independence Avenue SW
Washington, DC 20250

Administrator of the Environmental Protection Agency
Environmental Protection Agency
401 M Street SW
Washington, DC 20460

Secretary of Education
Department of Education
400 Maryland Avenue SW
Washington, DC 20202

Contact any school or library for the names and addresses of local elected representatives responsible for education.

In the United Kingdom, write to:

Minister of Health
Department of Health
Richmond House
79 Whitehall
London SW1A 2NS
England

Minister of Agriculture Fisheries and Food
Ministry of Agriculture Fisheries and Food
Whitehall Place
London SW1A 2HH
England

Minister of the Environment
Department of the Environment
2 Marsham Street
London SW1P 3EB
England

Minister of Education
Department of Education
Sanctuary Buildings
Great Smith Street
London SW1P 3BT
England

Contact any school or library for the names and addresses of local elected representatives responsible for education.

Public pressure is needed to force governments to do away with restriction and confinement of food animals in cages and crates. Write and express your concern about factory farming.

In Canada, write to:
Minister of Agriculture
House of Commons
Ottawa, Ontario
K1A 0A6

In the United States, write to:
Secretary of Agriculture
Department of Agriculture
14th Street and Independence Avenue SW
Washington, DC 20250

In the United Kingdom, write to:
Minister of Agriculture
Ministry of Agriculture Fisheries and Food
Whitehall Place
London SW1A 2HH

In 1990, the British government banned the existing type of white-veal calf pen. Since then it has been a punishable offense to keep a calf in a single pen unless the pen is wide enough to enable the calf to turn around easily. The calf must be given adequate dietary iron to maintain it in full health and vigor and, from two weeks of age, must be given enough fibrous food for the proper maintenance of the rumen.[1] The British government will soon introduce regulations to ban sow and tether stalls by the end of 1998.

Following the British example, a bill was introduced to the U.S. House of Representatives with similar proposals for reform. To date it has not been passed. Pressure is needed from taxpayers to ensure that bills similar to the ones in the U.K. are passed in the U.S. and in Canada.

Letters need not be long or complicated. Government officials know about the issue. If they don't, they will research it and find out. In your letter, you can say that you are aware of the many risks to human health caused by a meat-centered diet and of the enormous cost to taxpayers of treating illnesses such as heart attacks, strokes, and cancer. Point out that livestock farming inflicts immense damage on the environment.

State your opposition to the mistreatment, restriction, and confinement of factory-farm animals and the use of hormones, stimulants, tranquillizers, and antibiotics to control disease in the overcrowded pens. Point out that in consuming the flesh of these animals, people are also consuming an assortment of powerful drugs.

Ask that your letter be answered (it will be, as voters' comments are rarely ignored). Beware of misleading replies. Response letters are often cleverly worded to give an impression that the animals live under ideal conditions. The excuses will be many and worded in ways that seem to make sense. But you know the facts.

Tell the government to do everything in its power to bring an end to these cruel systems of restriction and to ensure that every farm animal has the freedom to be able, at the very least, to turn around, groom itself, get up, lie down, and stretch its limbs without difficulty.[2] Demand that these animals be given a diet appropriate in quality and quantity for their kind.

Ask your government to stop tax-supported research and development of factory-farm systems. Suggest that public funding be used instead to further the transition to growing vegetables, grains, and fruit organically.

Encourage state and provincial legislators to review the effectiveness of local laws protecting livestock in transit. If no such measures exist in your area, urge lawmakers to introduce them. Let them know that, as a taxpayer, you want laws passed because codes of practice are not good enough; codes are nothing more than suggested guidelines and in many cases are not adhered to or enforced. Suggest that animals in transit be given food and water during long hauls and that injured or sick animals be humanely destroyed at inspection points rather than returned to the point of origin, which may be hundreds of miles away. Suggest that unannounced government inspections of transport and slaughter facilities be routine, not rare.

Ask your member of parliament or congressional representative to support the banning of crates and battery cages. Suggest that intensive factory farming methods be raised as an election issue.

Copies of your letters should be sent to local humane societies and animal welfare organizations, editors of local newspapers, and producers at radio and television stations.

Writing to Businesses

Ask major fast-food chains to introduce veggie burgers and other alternatives to meat. Suggest that they accommodate the growing number of non-meat eaters. Tell them that salad bars are great but that there are also many other tasty fast-food meatless products available. Urge them to offer non-meat items for a trial period, and say that the results will speak for themselves.

The following addresses are the head offices of the world's largest fast-food chains:

McDonald's Restaurants of Canada Ltd.
McDonald's Place
Toronto, ON, Canada M3C 3L4

McDonald's Corporation
1 McDonald's Place
Oak Brook, IL 60521

McDonald'S U.K.
178-180 Edgeware Road
London, England W2 2DS

Wendy's
6715 Airport Road
Suite 301
Mississauga, ON, Canada L4V 1X2

Wendy's International Inc.
4288 W. Dublin
Granville Road, P.O. Box 256
Dublin, OH 43017-1442

M. & W. LTD (Wendy's)
3739 Cheval Place
London, England SW7 1EW

Burger King
201 City Centre Drive
8th Floor
Mississauga, ON, Canada L5B 2T4

Burger King
17777 Old Cutler Road
Miami, FL 33157

Burger King
20 Kew Road
2nd Floor
Richmond, Surrey, England TW9 2NA

Speak or write to the managers of local restaurants and grocery stores and ask them to start carrying a selection of vegetarian items. Let them know that many people no longer eat meat and that it is good business to consider those customers.

Join Animal Welfare Organizations

A good way to keep informed about animal issues is to contact animal welfare organizations and request membership information and campaign literature. Annual membership fees are usually modest.

Information from the organizations can be used to inform local media people, friends, neighbors, and co-workers about the issue. Contact the media in your area and suggest that they run programs and write articles on the issue of factory farming.

Bring children up as vegetarians. Many animal welfare organizations have material suitable for children and teens. Educate your children about the mistreatment of food animals and the advantages of a vegetarian diet. Don't let teachers go unchallenged when they present the make-believe world of happy farm animals. Volunteer an hour of your time to speak to a class about the issue. Use information from animal welfare organizations for reference material.

Speak Out against Cruelty: Silence Speaks for Itself!

Alert your family, friends, and coworkers that raising food animals affects the environment and our health. Encourage people to cut down and eliminate meat and animal products from their diets. Suggest that they visit health food stores to find good vegetarian products.

If you hear ridicule or criticism of the animal welfare movement, you can politely but firmly defend the validity of concern for animals. Point out that the circle of compassion does not start and end with people but should extend to all living creatures that share the earth. Briefly acquaint people with the facts or recommend that they read about the issue, as many people are not aware of the suffering these animals endure and that such barbaric practices are taking place legally.

When speaking out against the inhumane system of restriction, be factual and unemotional. It's less threatening to others if you speak about your own growing awareness of the mistreatment of farm animals and how you've changed your eating habits because of what you've learned. Don't attack meat eaters; talk about your own response to learning about the cruelty of factory farms.

As a community volunteer, you can organize forums and speak at club meetings, church groups, and service groups. Make these meetings interesting and informative by handing out leaflets on factory farming and vegetarianism. Provide meatless recipes and samples of vegetarian food. Ask a local vegetarian or health food store to sponsor your effort and perhaps supply food samples and information pamphlets on the issue.

CHAPTER 6

Vegetarian Organizations in Canada, the United States, and the United Kingdom

Vegetarian organizations are a great source of support for seasoned as well as new vegetarians. Many local vegetarian organizations have newsletters and educational material suitable for parents and teachers and organize recipe exchanges, monthly dinner events, annual food fairs, vegetarian restaurant discounts, and holiday season get-togethers. Some organizations have volunteer physicians and nutritionists on staff who give information on health-related issues. National organizations sponsor lectures and symposiums that feature guest speakers on animal-related issues, the environment, and, of course, vegetarianism.

The following list of local and national vegetarian societies was compiled with the assistance of the American Vegan Society, Malaga, New Jersey, and the Vegetarian Resource Group, Baltimore, Maryland.

Vegetarian Organizations in Canada

The Canadian Natural Hygiene Society
P.O. Box 235, Station T
Toronto, ON M6B 4A1

Carleton University Vegetarian Club
401 Unicenter Building
Ottawa, ON K1S 5B4

EarthSave Canada, Toronto Branch
3 Fermanagh Avenue
Toronto, ON M6R 1M1

EarthSave Canada, Vancouver Branch
P.O. Box 34277, Station D
Vancouver, BC V6J 4N8

Forest City Vegetarian Association
30 Buttermere Road
London, ON N6G 4L1

Hamilton Vegetarian Association
74 Alpine Avenue
Hamilton, ON L9A 1A6

Jewish Vegetarian Society of Toronto
113 Balliol Street
Toronto, ON M4S 1C2

Kitchener-Waterloo Vegetarian Association
285 Erb Street West, Suite 505
Waterloo, ON N2L 1W5

Lower Mainland Vegetarians
660 West 24th Avenue
Vancouver, BC V6Z 2B6

Ottawa Vegetarian Society
P.O. Box 4477, Station E
Ottawa, ON K1S 5B4

Toronto Vegetarian Society
736 Bathurst Street
Toronto, ON M5S 2R4

Vancouver Island Vegetarian Association
9675 5th Street
Sidney, BC V8L 2W9

Vegetarians of Alberta
9211 72nd Street
Edmonton, AB T6B 1Y6

Vegetarian Society of New Brunswick
308 Edinburgh Street
Fredericton, NB E3B 2O9

Vegetarian Associations in the United States
Arizona
Jewish Vegetarians of Arizona
P.O. Box 32842
Phoenix, AZ 85064

Vegetarian Society of Sierra Vista
P.O. Box 3461
Sierra Vista, AZ 85636

California
Bay Area Jewish Vegetarians
303 Adams Street, #201
Oakland, CA 94610

California Vegetarian Association
P.O. Box 6213
Thousand Oaks, CA 91359

East Bay Vegetarians
6037 Claremont Avenue
Oakland, CA 94618

Fremont Vegetarians
4872 Creekwood Drive
Fremont, CA 94555

Los Angeles Vegetarian Association
279 South Beverly Drive, Suite 690
Beverly Hills, CA 90212

New Vegetarian News
131 Maureen Circle
Pittsburg, CA 94565

Orange County Vegetarian Network
P.O. Box 15191
Santa Ana, CA 92705

Peninsula Vegetarians
284 Margarita Avenue
Palo Alto, CA 94306

Sacramento Vegetarian Society
823 28th Street
Sacramento, CA 95816

Santa Cruz Vegetarians
P.O. Box 2302
Santa Cruz, CA 95063

San Francisco Vegetarian Society
1450 Broadway
San Francisco, CA 94109

South Bay Vegetarians
260 Brooklyn Avenue
San Jose, CA 95128

South Valley Vegetarians
13810 Sheila Avenue
Morgan Hill, CA 95037

Vegan Resources
P.O. Box 2124
Orange, CA 92669

Vegetarian Inclined People (VIP)
1351 Royal Way, #33
San Luis Obispo, CA 93405

Vegetarian Singles
254 El Dorado Drive
Pacifica, CA 94044

Vegetarian Society
P.O. Box 34427
Los Angeles, CA 90034

Vegetarian Society, Inc.
2401 Lincoln Boulevard
Santa Monica, CA 90405

Colorado
Vegetarian Society of Colorado
P.O. Box 6773
Denver, CO 80206
(Branches in Boulder, Colorado Springs, Denver, Durango,
   Evergreen, Fort Collins, and Grand Junction)

Vegetarian Union of North America
P.O. Box 6853
Denver, CO 80206

Connecticut
New Haven Vegetarian Society
P.O. Box 1967
New Haven, CT 06509-19067

The Veggies (Teen Group)
55 Southwood Drive
New Canaan, CT 06840
or
157 Weed Street
New Canaan, CT 06840

District of Columbia
Vegetarian Society of the District of Columbia
P.O. Box 4921
Washington, DC 20008

Friends Vegetarian Society of North America
P.O. Box 53354
Washington, DC 20009

Florida
American Natural Hygiene Society
P.O. Box 30630
Tampa, FL 33630

Better Living & Nutrition Society of West Palm Beach
707 Chillingworth Dr.
West Palm Beach, FL 33409

Black Rhino Vegetarian Society
Route 3, Box 292
American Beach, FL 32034

Greater Orlando Vegetarian Society
P.O. Box 2381
Goldenrod, FL 32733

Indian River Vegetarian Society
2435 Tecca Dr., Oliver Estates
New Smyrna Beach, FL 32168

Life Balancing Center
1950 Sandra Dr.
Clearwater, FL 33546

Vegetarians of South Florida
Environmental Center
Miami-Dade Community College
11011 S.W. 104th Street
Miami, FL 33176

Vegetarian Singles Group
16750 N.E. 10th Avenue
North Miami Beach, FL 32102

Vegetarian Society of North Miami
131 NE 175th Street
North Miami Beach, FL 33162

Georgia
Vegetarian Society of Georgia
P.O. Box 2164
Norcross, GA 30191

Hawaii
Vegetarian Society of Honolulu
P.O. Box 25233
Honolulu, HI 96825

Idaho
Idaho Vegetarian League
1222 Freeman Lane, Suite 188
Pocatello, ID 83201

Illinois
Chicago Vegetarian Society, Inc.
P.O. Box 6154
Evanston, IL 60204

International Non-Violence and Vegetarian Society
4039 Enfield Ave.
Skokie, IL 60076

Vegetarian Health Society
2154 West Madison
Bellwood, IL 60104

Vegetarians in Motion
P.O. Box 6943
Rockford, IL 61125

Indiana
Bloomington Vegetarians
P.O. Box 6851
Bloomington, IN 47403

Vegetarian Society of Indianapolis
30 East Georgia, #216
Indianapolis, IN 46204

Iowa
Des Moines Vegetarian Society
4989 SE 72nd Avenue
Carlisle, IA 50047

Vegetarian Society of Central Iowa
c/o Dorothy Lewis
Iowa State University
291 Durham Center
Ames, IA 50011
(Support group for students and community members)

Kentucky
Vegetarian Society of Louisville
9004 Admiral Drive
Louisville, KY 40229-1534

Vegetarian Support Group
3217 Pacanack Court
Lexington, KY 40515

Maryland
Vegetarian Education Network
P.O. Box 896
Bel Air, MD 21014

Jewish Vegetarians of North America
P.O. Box 1463
Baltimore, MD 21203

Vegetarian Resource Group
P.O. Box 1463
Baltimore, MD 21203

Jewish Vegetarian Society, Inc.
P.O. Box 5722
Baltimore, MD 21208-0722

Massachusetts
Berkshire Vegetarian Society
60 Luce Road
Williamstown, MA 01267

Boston Vegetarian Society
P.O. Box 1071
Cambridge, MA 02238-1071

Cape Cod Vegetarian Society
P.O. Box 243
Sagamore Beach, MA 02562

Vegetarian Information Service
P.O. Box 985
Pocasset, MA 02559

Minnesota
Vegetarian Information Service of Minnesota
5049 Thomas Avenue South
Minneapolis, MN 55410

Vegetarian Society of Southern Minnesota
P.O. Box 1225
Mankato, MN 56001

Nebraska
Nebraska Vegetarian Society
P.O. Box 4775
Lincoln, NE 68504

Nevada
Sierra Vegetarian Society
315 Clay, #7
Reno, NV 89501-1730

New Hampshire
Vegetarians of Merrimack Valley
2 Morningside Drive
Nashua, NH 03060

New Jersey
American Vegan Society
501 Old Harding Highway
Malaga, NJ 08328

Simply Delicious Natural Foods
234-A North Hook Road, P.O. Box 124
Pennsville, NJ 08070

South Jersey Vegetarian Society
P.O. Box 272
Marlton, NJ 08053

Two Fu Vegetarian Singles Connection
P.O. Box 824
Westwood, NJ 07675

New Mexico
Vegetarian Society of Santa Fe
1007 Camino del Gusto
Santa Fe, NM 87505

New York
International Jewish Vegetarian Society
P.O. Box 144
Hurleyville, NY 12747

Island Vegetarians
P.O. Box 597
Lindenhurst, NY 11757

New York Vegan Society
6309 108th Street, #3A
Forest Hill, NY 11375

North American Vegetarian Society (NAVS)
P.O. Box 72
Dolgeville, NY 13329

Rochester Area Vegetarian Society
P.O. Box 37
Pittsford, NY 14534

Vegadine
(The Association of Vegetarian Dieticians and Nutrition Educators)
3835 Star Route 414
Burdett, NY 14818

Vegetarian Activist Collective/Women and Animal Activist Archives
184 Seeley St.
Brooklyn, NY 11218

Vegetarian Singles
P.O. Box 20304
New York, NY 10025

Vegetarian Society of Queens
15039 75 Avenue, #2A
Flushing, NY 11367

Whole Life Center
665 East 181 Street, 7A, Apt. 2
Bronx, NY 10457

North Carolina
Jewish Vegetarian Society
1310 LeClair Street
Chapel Hill, NC 27514

Mecklenberg Vegetarian Association
7302 Lancashire Drive
Charlotte, NC 28227

Triangle Vegetarian Society
P.O. Box 3364C
Chapel Hill, NC 27515-3364

Vegetarian Society of the Lower Cape Fear
4926 Marlin Court
Wilmington, NC 28403

Very Vegetarian Society
620 Bellview Street
Winston-Salem, NC 27103-3502

Western North Carolina Vegetarian Society
P.O. Box 368
Cullowhee, NC 28723

Ohio
Cincinnati Vegetarian Society
2424 Beekman Street
Cincinnati, OH 45214

Fit for Life Study Group
12521 Indian Hollow Rd.
Grafton, OH 44044

Ohio State University Vegetarian Society
Box 41, Ohio Union
1739 North High Street
Columbus, OH 43210

Summit Vegetarian Society
807 Washington Avenue
Cuyahoga Falls, OH 44221

Vegetarian Club of Canton
6407 Woodmoor N.W.
Canton, OH 44718

Vegetarian Society of Greater Youngstown Area
1631 Price Road
Youngstown, OH 44509

Vegetarian Society of the Greater Dayton Area
P.O. Box 404
Engelwood, OH 45322

Vegetarian Society of Toledo and Northwest Ohio
2655 Calverton Road
Toledo, OH 43607

Oregon
Portland Vegetarians
P.O. Box 19521
Portland, OR 97219

Salem Vegetarians
6301 Culver Drive SE
Salem, OR 97301

Pennsylvania
Lehigh Valley Vegetarians
1035 Flexer Avenue
Allentown, PA 18103

Pittsburgh Vegetarian Society
P.O. Box 234
Glenshaw, PA 15116

Vegetarians of Philadelphia
P.O. Box 24353
Philadelphia, PA 19120

Vegetarian Society of Central Pennsylvania
P.O. Box 11066
State College, PA 16805-1066

Vegetarian Education Network
P.O. Box 3347
West Chester, PA 19380

Rhode Island
Rhode Island Vegetarian Society
P.O. Box 28514
Providence, RI 02908

South Carolina
South Carolina Vegetarian Society
P.O. Box 1093
Lexington, SC 29071

Tennessee
Country Life Vegetarian Buffet/Prevention Clinic
1919 Division
Nashville, TN 37203

East Tennessee Vegetarian Society
P.O. Box 1974
Knoxville, TN 37901

Tennessee Vegetarian Society
P.O. Box 854
Knoxville, TN 37901

Texas
Austin Vegetarian Society
P.O. Box 2335
Cedar Park, TX 78613

Denton Area Vegetarian Organization
2040 West Oak
Denton, TX 76201

Houston Vegetarian Society
P.O. Box 770873
Houston, TX 77215

San Antonio Vegetarian and Humane Network
4115 E. Southcross Boulevard
San Antonio, TX 78222

San Antonio Vegetarian Society
P.O. Box 790391
San Antonio, TX 78279-0391

South Texas Vegetarian Society
P.O. Box 314
West Columbus, TX 77486

Texas Vegetarian Society
5416 Gurley Avenue
Dallas, TX 75223

Utah
Vegetarian Society of Utah
3678 East Millcreek Road
Salt Lake City, UT 84109

Vermont
Vermont Vegetarian Society
Rural Route 1, Box 1797
North Ferrisburg, VT 04573

Virginia
Vegetarian Society of New River Valley
117 South Main Street
Blackburg, VA 24060

Washington
Bodhi Vegetarian Society
1411 East Fir Street
Seattle, WA 98122-5531

Northwestern Coordinator for NAVS Affiliate Groups
P.O. Box 303
Burton, WA 98013

Spokane Vegetarian Society
4223 E. 26th Avenue
Spokane, WA 99223

Wisconsin
Vegan Action
P.O. Box 2701
Madison, WI 53701-2701

Vegetarian Society of the University of Wisconsin
2642-A North Bremen
Milwaukee, WI 53212

Vegetarian Organizations in the United Kingdom

English Vegan Society
123 Baker Street
Enfield, Middlesex EN1 5HA

London Vegans
7 Deansbrook Road
Edgeware, Middlesex HA8 9BE

The Vegan Society
7 Battle Road, St. Leonards-on-Sea
East Sussex TN37 7AA

The Vegan Way
47 Highlands Road
Leatherhead, Surrey KT22 8NQ

The Vegetarian Society (UK) or the Vegetarian Society Youth
  Section
Parkdale, Dunham Road
Altrincham, Cheshire WA14 4QG

Veggies
180 Mansfield Road
Nottingham NG1 3HU

Welsh Vegan
9 Mawddwy Cottages
Minllyn, Dinas Mawddwy
Machynlleth, Wales SY20 9LW

CHAPTER 7

Animal Welfare Organizations in Canada, the United States, and the United Kingdom

Animal Welfare Organizations in Canada

Animal Alliance of Canada
1640 Bayview Avenue, Suite 1916
Toronto, ON M4G 4E9

Animal Defense League of Canada
P.O. Box 3880, Station C
Ottawa, ON K1Y 4M5

Ark II
P.O. Box 687, Station Q
Toronto, ON M4T 2N5

Canadians for Ethical Treatment of Food Animals
Box 35597, Station E
Vancouver, BC V6M 4G9

Canadian Vegans for Animal Rights (C-VAR)
620 Jarvis Street, Suite 2504
Toronto, ON M4Y 2R8

Humane societies—check local telephone directories for listings

Intensive Farming Review
P.O. Box 1721, Station A
Vancouver, BC V6C 2P7

Manitoba Animal Alliance
P.O. Box 3193
Winnipeg, MB R3C 0K2

World Society for the Protection of Animals
55 University Avenue, Suite 902
Toronto, ON M5J 2H7

Animal Welfare Organizations in the United States

Action for Animals
P.O. Box 20184
Oakland, CA 94620

Adopt-a-Cow
Rd. 1, Box 839
Port Royal, PA 17082

Advocates for Animals
96 Fisher Hill Road
Cheshire, MA 01225

The American Vegan Society
501 Old Harding Highway
Malaga, NJ 08328

Animal Place
3448 Laguna Creek Trail
Vacaville, CA 95688-9724

Animal Rights Mobilization (ARM)
P.O. Box 6989
Denver, CO 80206

The Animals' Crusaders
2015 Hoyt Avenue
Everett, WA 98201

Animal Welfare Institute
P.O. Box 3650
Washington, DC 20007

Citizens for Humane Farming
P.O. Box 27
Cambridge, MA 02238

Coalition to End Animal Suffering and Exploitation (CEASE)
P.O. Box 27
Cambridge, MA 02238

EarthSave Foundation
706 Frederick Street
Santa Cruz, CA 95062

Farm Animal Reform Movement
P.O. Box 30654
Bethesda, MD 20824

Farm Animal Sanctuary
P.O. Box 150
Watkins Glen, NY 14891

The Farm Animals
P.O. Box 33086
Cleveland, OH 44133

Food Animals Concerns Trust (FACT)
P.O. Box 14599
Chicago, IL 60614

Friends of Animals
P.O. Box 1244
Norwalk, CT 06856

Humane Farming Association
Suite #6, 1550 California Street
San Francisco, CA 94109

Humane societies—check local telephone directories for listings

Humane Society of the United States (HSUS)
2100-L Street N.W.
Washington, DC 20037

International Society for Animal Rights
421 South State Street
Clarks Summit, PA 18411

Iowa Alliance for Animals
P.O. Box 1263
Welch Ave. Station
Ames, IA 50010

Jews for Animal Rights
255 Humphrey Street
Marblehead, MA 01945

Mobilization for Animals
P.O. Box 1679
Columbus, OH 43216

New Hampshire Animal Rights League
Bean Hill Road
Northfield, NH 03276

People for Animal Rights
P.O. Box 2928
Olathe, KS 66062

People for the Ethical Treatment of Animals (PETA)
P.O. Box 42516
Washington, DC 20015

Physicians' Committee for Responsible Medicine
P.O. Box 6322
Washington, DC 20015

Progressive Animal Welfare Society (PAWS)
15305 44th Avenue West, P.O. Box 1037
Lynnwood, WA 98046

Society for Animal Protective Legislation
P.O. Box 3719, Georgetown Station
Washington, DC 20007

Trans-Species Unlimited
P.O. Box 1351
State College, PA 16804

United Animal Defenders
P.O. Box 33086
Cleveland, OH 44133

United Poultry Concerns
P.O. Box 59367
Potomac, MD 20859

Washtenaw Citizens for Animal Rights
P.O. Box 2614
Ann Arbor, MI 48106

Web of Life
P.O. Box 2124
Orange, CA 92669

Animal Welfare Organizations in the United Kingdom

Advocates for Animals
10 Queensferry Street
Edinburgh, Scotland EH2 4PG

Animal Aid
7 Castle Street
Tonbridge, Kent TN9 1BH

Animal Concern (Scotland)
62 Dumbarton Road
Glasgow, G3 8RE

Animal Concern Today
P.O. Box 67
Plymouth, PL1 1TH

Animals' Vigilantes
James Mason House, 24 Salisbury Street
Fordingbridge, Hants. SP6 1AF

Ark Campaigns
498 Harrow Road
London, W9 3QA

The Athene Trust
20 Lavant Street
Petersfield, Hants., GU32 3EW

Chicken's Lib
P.O. Box 2
Holmsfirth, Huddersfield, HD7 1QT

Compassion in World Farming
20 Lavant Street
Petersfield, Hants., GU32 3EW

Dartmoor Livestock Protection Society
Crooked Meadow, Stidston Lane
South Brent, Devon, TQ10 3JS

The Farm and Food Society
4 Willifield Way
London, NW11 7XT

Fight Against Animal Cruelty in Europe (FAACE)
19A Stanley Street
Southport, Merseyside, PR9 0BY

The Free Range Egg Association
37 Tanza Road
London NW3 2UA

The Movement for Compassionate Living
47 Highland Road
Leatherhead, Surrey, KT22 8NQ

Quaker Concern for Animal Welfare
Webb's Cottage, Woolpits Road
Saling, Braintree, Essex, CM7 5DZ

Royal Society for the Prevention of Cruelty to Animals (RSPCA)
Causeway
Horsham, West Sussex, RH12 1HG

Students Campaign for Animal Rights (SCAR)
Mandela Building, 99 Oxford Road,
Manchester

Universities Federation for Animal Welfare
8 Hamilton Close
Potters Bar, Herts., EN6 3QD

Notes

Chapter 2. Vegetarianism for Good Health

1. *Vegetarianism in a Nutshell* (Baltimore, MD: Vegetarian Resource Group).
2. *Animal Rights* (Lynnwood, PA: Progressive Animal Welfare Society).
3. Neal Barnard, M.D., "Eating For Life," *People for the Ethical Treatment of Animals News* 1, no. 8.
4. *Keeping a Healthy Heart* (Washington, D.C.: People for the Ethical Treatment of Animals).
5. *The Dire Effects of a Meat-Based Diet on Human Health* (Ames, IA: Iowa Alliance for Animals).
6. "Relations of Meat, Fat, and Fiber Intake to the Risk of Colon Cancer in a Prospective Study Among Women," *New England Journal of Medicine*, 13 December 1990: 1664.
7. Neal Barnard, M.D., "Eating For Life," *People for the Ethical Treatment of Animals News* 1, no. 8.
8. *The Vegetarian Option for Ethical Reasons* (Ottawa, ON: Animal Defence League of Canada, 1985), 3.
9. *The New Four Food Groups* (Washington, D.C.: Physicians' Committee for Responsible Medicine), 7.
10. Lynn Thomas, *Animal Factories in Canada* (Toronto, ON: Toronto Humane Society, 1986), 32.
11. Ibid., 32, 33.
12. *Consumer Alert* (Petersfield, England: Compassion in World Farming).
13. "Food: Scrambled. After 2,000 Poisoning Cases, Fear of Salmonella Is No Yolk," *Time Magazine*, 13 May 1991.
14. "Consumer Alert," *New Scientist Magazine*, 3 May 1987.
15. "Salmonella Poisoning Kills 61," *Agscene Magazine*, no. 102 (Spring 1991): 7.
16. Intensive Farming Review, *Factsheet 17* (January 1990).
17. *Veterinary Record*, no. 5 (September 1987).
18. *The Vealer Magazine*, April 1984.

19. *Fact Sheet: Perception and Facts on Veal Production* (Mississauga, ON: Ontario Farm Animal Council).
20. *Fact Sheet: Questions and Answers about Veal* (Washington, D.C.: Humane Society of the United States).
21. Ibid.
22. *Fact Sheet: Perception and Facts on Veal Production* (Mississauga, ON: Ontario Farm Animal Council).
23. *Cancer-Causing Chemicals in Foods* (Report), Committee of Interstate and Foreign Commerce, 1979.
24. *Problems in Preventing the Marketing of Raw Meat and Poultry Containing Potentially Harmful Residue* (Washington, D.C.: Comptroller General of the U.S., April 1979).
25. Tina Harrison, "Is Meat Hazardous to Your Health?," *Toronto Star*, 4 October 1990.
26. Lynn Thomas, *Animal Factories in Canada* (Toronto, ON: Toronto Humane Society, 1986), 19.
27. Ibid.
28. Jeanne Mayer and Joanna Dwyer, "Food For Thought," *North American Vegetarian Society Newsletter.*
29. "Cold Remedies: What Works and What Doesn't," *University of California at Berkeley Wellness Letter* 8, no. 5 (February 1992).
30. *Agribusiness Exposed* (Toronto, ON: Canadian Vegans For Animal Rights).
31. Lynn Thomas, *Animal Factories in Canada* (Toronto, ON: Toronto Humane Society, 1986), 19.
32. Ibid.
33. "The New Four Food Groups," *Physicians' Committee for Responsible Medicine Update*, May/June 1991.
34. Neal Barnard, M.D., *The Power of Your Plate: A Plan for Better Living* (Summertown, TN: Book Publishing Company, 1990).

Chapter 3. Vegetarianism for the Benefit of Animals

1. Lynn Thomas, *Animal Factories in Canada* (Toronto, ON: Toronto Humane Society, 1986), 5.
2. *New Scientist Magazine*, 16 September 1989.
3. "Torture in North America," *Front Line News* (San Francisco, CA: Humane Farming Association), no. 4 (Spring 1988).
4. *The Dangers of Factory Farming* (San Francisco, CA: Humane Farming Association).
5. Konrad Lorenz, "Comments on Battery Hens and Those Who Practice It," *Das Tier* (*The Animal*), February 1976.
6. *"Torture in North America,"* *Front Line News* (San Francisco, CA: Humane Farming Association), no. 4 (Spring 1988).
7. *Fact Sheet on Broiler Chickens* (Washington, D.C.: Humane Society of the United States).
8. *Factory Farming* (Cleveland, OH: United Animal Defenders), 3.
9. *Intensive Egg, Chicken and Turkey Production* (Huddersfield, England: Chicken's Lib), 17.
10. Ibid., 20.
11. Intensive Farming Review, *Newsletter Number 1* (January 1988).
12. *Slaughter of Red Meat Animals* (Petersfield, England: Compassion in World Farming), 8.
13. *Poultry World Magazine*, February 1990.
14. Ibid.
15. *Chicken Meat Production, Can You Face the Facts?* (Huddersfield, England: Chicken's Lib).
16. Ibid.
17. Ibid.
18. Ibid.
19. *Meet the Milk Producers* (Williamsport, PA: Transpecies Unlimited).
20. Robert B. Thomas, *The Old Farmer's Almanac, 1991, Special Canadian Edition*, 199th ed. (Dublin, NH: Yankee Publishing, 1990).
21. *New Scientist Magazine*, January 1972.

22. *Report of the Bramwell Committee* (H.M. Stationery Office, 1965).
23. "1987 Report of the Expert Committee on Farm Animal Welfare and Behaviour in Canada," *Farm Welfare in Canada: Issues and Priorities* (1987): 5.
24. *Information on Factory Farming* (Cleveland, OH: United Animal Defenders).
25. Nancy E. Wiswall, *The Production of Veal as an Animal Welfare Issue* (Washington, D.C.: Humane Society of the United States).
26. *Report of the Bramwell Committee* (H.M. Stationery Office, 1965).
27. *Information on Factory Farming* (Cleveland, OH: United Animal Defenders).
28. Nancy E. Wiswall, *The Production of Veal as an Animal Welfare Issue* (Washington, D.C.: Humane Society of the United States).
29. Ibid.
30. Ibid.
31. Humane Society of the United States, *Fact Sheet on Beef.*
32. United Animal Defenders, *Information on Factory Farming.*
33. Richard A. Battaglia and Vernon B. Mayrose, *Handbook of Livestock Management Techniques* (Minneapolis, MN: Burgess, 1981).
34. United Animal Defenders, *Information on Factory Farming.*
35. "The Petersons Talk about Pastureland Pigs," *Quarterly Publication of the Animal Welfare Institute*, Fall/Winter 1989-1990: 10-12.
36. *Meet Your Meat* (Williamsport, PA: Transpecies Unlimited).
37. B. Sommer, H. H. Sambraus, H. Krausslich, "Study Submitted to the World Federation for the Protection of Animals," *Factory Farming: The Experiment that Failed* (Washington, D.C.: Animal Welfare Institute, 1987), 47.
38. *Does Confinement Cause Distress in Sows* (The Athene Trust).
39. "The Petersons Talk about Pastureland Pigs," *Quarterly Publication of the Animal Welfare Institute*, Fall/Winter 1989-1990: 10-12.

40. Ibid.

41. Ibid.

42. *Factory Farming* (Cleveland, OH: United Animal Defenders), 1.

43. "The Petersons Talk about Pastureland Pigs," *Quarterly Publication of the Animal Welfare Institute*, Fall/Winter 1989-1990: 10-12.

44. Temple Grandin, "Mechanical, Electrical and Anesthetic Stunning Methods for Livestock," *International Journal for the Study of Animal Problems* (1980).

45. Ibid.

46. *Think Before You Eat* (Toronto, ON: Toronto Vegetarian Society); further information obtained in conversation with this group. Compassion in World Farming, "CIWF Investigates Slaughter in Spain," *Agscene Magazine* 102 (Spring 1991): 22-23.

47. Lynn Thomas, *Animal Factories in Canada* (Toronto, ON: Toronto Humane Society, 1986), 8.

48. "Humane Pre-slaughter Bill Could Turn Violators into Criminals," *Washington Star*, 21 July 1978.

49. Ibid.

50. "Intensive Farming Review," *Meat Processing Magazine* (February 1989).

51. Danielle Crittenden, "Agony Before Death," *Toronto Sun*, 17 October 1982.

52. *Ritual Slaughter: Shechitah* (Cleveland, OH: The Farm Animal).

53. Phyllis Klasky Karas, "Is Kosher Slaughtering Inhumane?," *Moment Magazine*, February 1991.

54. *Ritual Slaughter: Shechitah* (Cleveland, OH: The Farm Animal).

55. Temple Grandin, "Humanitarian Aspects of Shechitah in the United States," *Judaism: A Quarterly Journal of Jewish Life and Thought*, Fall 1990.

56. Ibid.

57. Peter C. Lovenheim, "Kosher Slaughter" (paper), April 1983.

58. Temple Grandin, "Humanitarian Aspects of Shechitah in the United States," *Judaism: A Quarterly Journal of Jewish Life and Thought*, Fall 1990.
59. Temple Grandin, letter to the author, 17 July 1991, and telephone interviews.

Chapter 4. Vegetarianism for a Healthier Environment

1. *Vegetarianism Like It Is* (Washington, D.C.: Vegetarian Information Services).
2. Frances Moore Lappé, *Diet for a Small Planet*, rev. ed. (New York: Ballantine, 1975), 10.
3. Lynn Thomas, *Animal Factories in Canada* (Toronto, ON: Toronto Humane Society, 1986), 36.
4. *Solstice Magazine* (December/January 1989).
5. *Factory Farming* (Cleveland, OH: United Animal Defenders).
6. Ellie Kirzner, *Now Magazine: Toronto's Weekly News* 7, no. 16, 23 December 1987–6 January 1988.
7. Lynn Thomas, *Animal Factories in Canada* (Toronto, ON: Toronto Humane Society, 1986), 14.
8. *Vegetarian Living* (Washington, D.C.: People for the Ethical Treatment of Animals).
9. "Meatfacts," *Vegetarian Voice Magazine* 15, (1989).
10. Vistara Parnham, *What's Wrong with Eating Meat?* (Corona, NY: Ananda Marga Publications, 1979), 40.

Chapter 5. Writing Letters to Encourage Change

1. *Information Sheet: Proposed Legislation* (Vancouver, BC: Intensive Farming Review).
2. *Help! Stop the Suffering* (Petersfield, England: Compassion in World Farming).

Recommended reading...

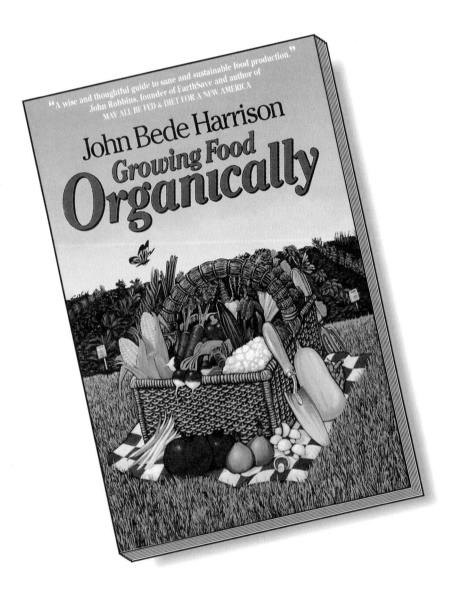

"A wise and thoughtful guide to sane and sustainable food production."
John Robbins, founder of EarthSave and author of
MAY ALL BE FED & DIET FOR A NEW AMERICA

John Bede Harrison

Growing Food Organically